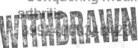

C O N Q U E R I N G

Rheumatoid Arthritis

CONQUERING

Rheumatoid Arthritis

THE LATEST BREAKTHROUGHS AND TREATMENTS

THOMAS F. LEE, Ph.D.

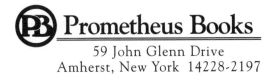

Prometheus Books

59 John Glenn Drive
Amherst, New York 14228-2197

Published 2001 by Prometheus Books

Inquiries should be addressed to
Prometheus Books
59 John Glenn Drive
Amherst, New York 14228-2197
VOICE: 716-691-0133, ext. 207
FAX: 716-564-2711
WWW.PROMETHEUSBOOKS.COM

08 07 06 05   9 8 7 6

Library of Congress Cataloging-in-Publication Data

Lee, Thomas F.
    Conquering rheumatoid arthritis : the latest breakthoughs and treat-
ments / Thomas F. Lee.
        p. cm.
    Includes bibliographical references and index.
    ISBN 1-57392-886-0 (pbk. : alk. paper)
    1. Rheumatoid arthritis—Popular works. I. Title.

RC933 .L43 2001
616.7'227—dc21

                                                        2001016111

Printed in the United States of America on acid-free paper

Contents

Contents

Acknowledgments

I offer heartfelt thanks to my wife, Eileen, and my children, Anne, Brian, Emily, Julie, Bridget, and Rebecca, for their generous support and encouragement. I am very grateful to Linda Greenspan Regan for her careful and helpful editing; to my talented student, Sean Horrigan, for his illustrations; and to my rheumatologist, Dr. John Yost, whose advice and care is deeply appreciated.

Preface

In 1882, while returning from a trip to Italy, forty-one-year-old Pierre-Auguste Renoir was surprised and alarmed when he experienced the first puzzling attack of piercing pain in his joints accompanied by a feeling of crushing fatigue. He was no doubt relieved as these first symptoms abated. However, the renowned French impressionist artist, in the prime of his life, whose enthusiasm was so vividly reflected in the vibrant colors and textures of his paintings, already had unwittingly entered a world of inexorable progressive disability.

Over the next twenty years Renoir continued with his beloved painting despite the crippling swelling gradually developing in his knuckles, fingers, knees, and feet. His physicians, true to the ignorance of their time, prescribed enemas and fever medications that were of little help. By 1903 the disease became more aggressive and Renoir was now barely able to walk or even sit before a canvas, painting with the brush wedged into his hands. Aided by a supportive family and fierce determination he persisted in his work, and was carried to his easel every morning. He died of pneumonia at seventy-eight, having painted for several hours that very evening.

We now know that the courageous artist, despite his iron

will and the best efforts of his physicians, had been forced to live much of his life in the grip of rheumatoid arthritis (RA), a disease that has plagued millions of humans for thousands of years.

The earliest known appearance of rheumatoid arthritis is in sixty-five-hundred-year-old skeletal remains of Native Americans—long before French physician Augustin-Jacob Landre-Beauvais published the first clinical description of the disease symptoms in 1800. In Renoir's day the common condition was often referred to as "rheumatic gout" even though in 1858 British physician Alfred B. Garrod had already coined the term "rheumatoid arthritis" to distinguish the disease from gout, an unrelated chemical disorder in which uric acid crystals form painful deposits in the joints.

This is not to imply that even today the signs and symptoms of rheumatoid arthritis are immediately recognizable or that the diagnosis is readily made, or especially not that the progression and severity of the disease are the same in all individuals—quite the contrary. More on that later, but first—what is the purpose of this book?

✚   ✚   ✚

In 1995 I was diagnosed with rheumatoid arthritis. One of my varied reactions to this unwelcome news was similar to that of the great Samuel Johnson, the eighteenth-century author of the first comprehensive dictionary of the English language, when he was asked about his attitude toward his mortality. "The thought of death," replied Johnson in one of his more famous understatements, "concentrates the mind wonderfully."

The thought of my life with RA certainly had that effect on me. As a biologist, researcher, professor, and author of earlier books on disease-related topics, my professional interests easily merged with my personal desire to find out more about my new, painful companion. I wanted to know the options open to me and to the millions of others confronted with this disease. I knew that there were medications available to alleviate some of the pain and inflammation. Would these dampen the fire but not put it out? Was there any hope for more powerful remedies for the discomfort and damage inflicted by this disease? Quite frankly, what about the possibility of an actual cure, a way to make this just go away and not come back?

I already had written about many awesome developments in molecular biology, genetics, and biotechnology and their application to medicine, which were already well underway in this transition between the twentieth century and the new millennium. To my relief I discovered that many of these insights now are being applied to the fight against RA and related diseases.

Specifically, scientists are making significant progress in understanding the intricate workings of the immune system, that marvelous complex of cells and chemicals that protects our bodies from foreign invaders such as viruses, bacteria, or parasites. In RA this immune system, for reasons as yet unknown, turns against the very body that houses it and begins a pattern of painful, progressive inflammation and damage, particularly in the joints.

Why does this happen? What turns on this powerful immune system to attack us and what can be done to turn it off? The answers to those questions may turn out to be simple but the road to finding them has posed a challenge.

Scientists know, for example, that a person's genetic makeup can play an important role in susceptibility to RA. The surface of the white blood cells of about 65 percent of people with RA share a common inherited characteristic, a "genetic marker" that signals that the bearer of the gene for that marker faces a future of more severe arthritis than those without the gene. However, individuals without the marker can still develop RA, and many with this marker never experience the disease. Moreover, susceptibility to RA is probably polygenic; that is, it develops under the influence of an as yet unknown number of genes influenced by nongenetic or environmental factors.

A massive, coordinated effort is underway to find all the genetic factors that predispose some to RA as well as those genes that are connected with disease severity. The National Institutes of Health (NIH) and the Arthritis Foundation have joined forces to support the North American Rheumatoid Arthritis Consortium. We will explain the work of this partnership of twelve research centers across the United States, which is a valuable resource for genetic studies of RA.

This research is by no means limited to the United States, but is an international effort. For example, in 1999 scientists at the Weizmann Institute in Rehovot, Israel, discovered a gene responsible for creating a protein that could help block RA as well as diabetes and muscular dystrophy.

We'll also look at the exciting possibilities of gene therapy. Experiments with putting genes into people have in some cases shown promise toward correcting a wide range of problems with genetic roots, including cancer, diabetes, and now RA.

In the search for what might trigger the onset of RA, researchers have investigated hundreds of microbes—bacteria, viruses, and others—without as yet being able to pinpoint any specific one as a cause of RA. The search goes on, as we shall see. In a real sense it would be ideal if we could home in on one infectious agent responsible for RA, for then it might offer the hope for a vaccine.

We will look at the ongoing search for answers to these and many other puzzling questions about RA. Medical science has always approached these kinds of questions by first analyzing the workings of the particular body system under attack and then looking for the key steps in that system that might be promising points at which to intervene. By locating the right points, scientists might be able to control the disease process. Familiar examples of such successful control of other diseases are numerous.

We have discovered that the chemical insulin regulates the entrance of sugar into our cells. Because we learned also that the diabetic pancreas is deficient in producing insulin we can control the sugar levels in the blood of a person with diabetes through life-saving insulin injections.

Or, now that we understand how certain white blood cells in the immune system make protective antibodies in response to foreign substances entering the body, we have modified the tetanus bacteria so that they are too weak to cause the fatal infection of tetanus, but are still able to set off a massive buildup of protective antibodies when injected as a vaccine beneath our skin. Using the same principles, we now have effective vaccines against diphtheria, whooping cough, polio, measles, and other devastating diseases that once swept through human populations unchecked.

To find out what causes RA and how to improve our control over it, our immune system is now under intense scrutiny, aided by powerful research tools that can peer into our cells and even into the molecules inside and surrounding those cells. Our growing understanding has already paid dividends—during the period between 1998 and 1999 the U.S. Food and Drug Administration (FDA) approved five new, innovative drugs to combat RA.

These new medications for those with RA are only the first to come from what is a new message of hope based on an expanding understanding of the intricate workings of the immune system, and consequently more effective ways to develop and deliver effective treatment. This book is the story of the unfolding of this exciting new era.

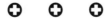

While the message of this book is one of hope for the future it is important for the reader to understand that even now, early diagnosis and prompt, appropriate treatment of RA can minimize joint and tissue damage and may have a profoundly beneficial effect on the course of the disease. While it is regrettably true that there is now no single chemical or therapy that can completely cure RA, medications are available, often in combination form, that can control pain and inflammation and assist in helping a person continue to work and maintain a desirable lifestyle.

Treatment is not confined to medications. It encompasses a variety of approaches depending on the severity of the disease, including exercise and physical therapy as well as emotional support for the person with RA and his/her family. The physician is central to this treatment. This book is not written to offer specific medical advice or to interfere in any way with the crucially important physician-client relationship, which is based on trust and confidence in the physician's competence and caring. On the contrary, it will support and encourage that relationship by helping the reader with RA to become a better-informed advocate as partner with his/her physician in the management of the disease.

Through personal experience I know that when one is diagnosed with a disease there is a natural tendency to want to know as much as possible about it, particularly and understandably with emphasis on what can be done to alleviate its symptoms, what can be done to reduce its effects on one's life, and, ideally, how it might be made to disappear.

The physician shares all of those goals. The physician-client partnership is essential in working out the most effective treatment regime for the individual. In those decisions, whether they involve RA or other diseases—such as cancer, diabetes, muscular dystrophy, or asthma—I am convinced that the individual deserves to be helped to be as knowledgeable as possible about the disease that may profoundly affect her and her family's lives. She should know the available treatments not just by name but also the way in which these medications may affect the disease process. This book will assist by guiding the reader through what can be a complicated and confusing search by translating the language of medical science into simpler terms along the way.

Beyond that it will assist you in understanding and following the ongoing development of the exciting new possibilities that enable us to comprehend and combat this disease, which has entered the lives of so many of us. In this age of the "Information Superhighway" there is a bewildering array of thousands of health-related Web sites on the Internet. Not all of the information and opinions available are accurate. This book will direct you to the most reliable Web sites dedicated to RA education and research. It will explain how one can keep track of, for example, new medications approved by the FDA, and it will describe how new drugs are developed and tested—first in the laboratory, then in animals, and finally in clinical trials with human volunteers. You will learn not only how you can find out about these clinical trials testing new therapies for RA, but also how it is possible to participate in those studies, if you so desire.

Right now the goals of RA therapy are to reduce pain and stiffness in the joints, control inflammation, prevent the destruction of joints, and support normal freedom of motion for as long as possible. No single medication can do that now, and it is likely—in the near future at least—that newer medications will be used as far more effective partners in that effort. While we cannot rule out the discovery of a "magic bullet" that will stop RA in its tracks, there is more optimism for the emergence of new pharmaceuticals that will block the reactions of RA at such critical crossroads that it will prevent the disease process from turning down the paths leading to pain, swelling, and damage.

This book will provide you with the sites of biotechnology companies and university and medical centers where cutting-edge research is now underway. Most important, it will give you the basic vocabulary needed to follow the progress of that research.

All of these recent and impending breakthroughs will be much more meaningful if we begin by looking at the basics of what we know about RA and our immune system while emphasizing the crucial questions which medical science is now beginning to answer.

CHAPTER 1

When Is
Arthritis Rheumatoid?

Many of our medical and scientific terms have Latin or Greek origins. The word *arthritis* is a combination of the Greek *arthron*, meaning joint, and *itis*, referring to *inflammation*. If you consider that *inflammare* is the Latin verb meaning "to set on fire," the word is an apt description of the location and sensation of the discomfort experienced by so many.

We'll have lots more to say about what goes on during the process of inflammation later because the search for new and better ways to deal with RA depends on an increased understanding and control of a complicated set of events. For now, let's emphasize the fact that normal inflammation is a natural and absolutely essential part of the body's immune or defense system. In other words, all of us periodically experience some inflammation as a result of, for example, a minor infection or perhaps a sprain.

Our first line of defense against foreign invaders—including viruses, bacteria, and fungi—is the skin and the moist mucous membranes that line our respiratory, reproductive, and digestive tracts. Unpleasant as it may seem, we are constantly bombarded by hordes of these invisible microscopic creatures. Some of them manage to make their way through the physical barrier of the skin or mucous membranes and enter deeper tissues. Think of what happens after the common experience of getting a splinter in your finger. A splinter almost always carries bacteria on it, and unless the splinter is removed quickly, the pierced area becomes red, swollen, painful, and even warm within a few hours. That is normal inflammation at work. We are very fortunate that this temporary discomfort is triggered, because otherwise the bacteria could multiply uncontrollably and result in a fatal infection.

In our tissues there is a resident population of wandering white blood cells—the *macrophages,* a name based on the Greek *phagein,* "to eat," and *makros,* "large." Macrophages are indeed big eaters. They can be considered as efficient trash collectors that grab onto and digest whatever debris or foreign particles they come across. When they encounter and engulf invaders from the outside world, such as bacteria from a splinter, the macrophages release chemicals that cause local blood vessels to leak fluid into the surrounding tissues, which gives rise to swelling. Vessels exiting the area become narrowed, promoting a buildup of blood, resulting in localized redness.

The macrophages also release chemicals that attract other specialized white blood cells to the area. These new arrivals join in the battle in various ways. The increased cellular chemical reactions (metabolism) in the irritated area generate warmth. Some of the released chemicals, along with the mounting pressure in the swelling tissues, incite painful sensations. All of this results in the classic signs of inflammation— pain, swelling, redness, and heat. When the invading agent has been exterminated, the inflammation subsides and disappears.

There are several important differences between this scenario resulting from a dirty splinter and the inflammation that occurs in RA. While much of the process is identical, the triggering event—that is, what sets off the inflammation in RA—is still unknown. It seems unlikely that there is one specific factor that accounts for all cases of RA. While the search goes on for bacteria or viruses that might play a role, RA is widely regarded by many as not one disease but rather a common response to what could be a number of different stimuli.

Also, in RA two of the types of white blood cells that answer the call of the macrophages, the *T cells* and *B cells,* somehow escape the controls that normally monitor and regulate their activities. They enter into a self-perpetuating cycle of inflammation and damage—the very heart of the problem in RA. They just keep on fighting when they should stop.

✛   ✛   ✛

Pain, stiffness, and often swelling are familiar symptoms of the more than one hundred forms of arthritis. Sometimes this discomfort may come from microorganisms such as bacteria, protozoa, viruses, or fungi that have invaded the body, sparking various forms of *infectious arthritis.* This may occur after wounds or surgery, or through Lyme disease, gonorrhea, or even tuberculosis. Please note that "infectious" does not mean that the disease can be transmitted from one person to another. It means that the condition is caused by a *pathogen,* in short, any disease-causing microorganism. Arthritis is not "catchable."

A form of RA occasionally occurs in people who also have *psoriasis,* a common scaling skin disorder. This type of arthritis, referred to as *psoriatic arthritis,* also often affects the joints at the ends of the fingers (not so in typical RA).

Most frequently arthritis takes the form of *osteoarthritis* (OA), from the Latin *os,* meaning "bone." Osteoarthritis is often referred to as *degenerative joint disease* (DJD). The smooth, moist, rubbery *cartilage,* which protects the ends of the bones at the joints, wears down and becomes thinner and rougher. If a substantial amount of cartilage wears away, the unprotected bones in the joint rub together, causing severe pain and reducing joint movement. This "wear-and-tear" of osteoarthritis, brought on by a variety of factors, including lack of exercise, obesity, overuse, joint injury, and aging, needs to be carefully distinguished from RA during diagnosis— although one can have both OA and RA simultaneously. OA affects more than 21 million Americans.

To label arthritis as "rheumatoid" is to indicate in a some-what roundabout way that this form of arthritis usually is marked by swelling in the inflamed joints. The Greek *rheuma* means a watery flow, so the early descriptions of the disease reflect the rather vague image of the swelling joints filling up with water.

Some general confusion over terminology is not unusual because there are more than one hundred diseases considered to be *rheumatic diseases*, only one of which is RA. The rheumatic diseases are those that affect *connective tissue*, par-ticularly within the joints and related structures such as bone. The many different forms of arthritis are just a part of the rheumatic disease spectrum. Other rheumatic diseases (see glossary) include *fibromyalgia, scleroderma, systemic lupus ery-thematosus* (also known as SLE and *lupus*), *ankylosing spondylitis*, and *polymyalgia rheumatica*.

How Common Is Arthritis?

More than 40 million Americans have some form of arthritis, costing the U.S. economy $65 billion per year in medical care and lost wages. Other societies are affected just as dramatically. In Canada arthritis affects one in every five adults and is the leading cause of long-term disability. In the United Kingdom, 8 million people have arthritis, which accounts for one-fifth of all visits to physicians. According to the Arthritis Foundation of Ireland 13 percent of the Irish show some signs of arthritis.

Rheumatoid arthritis afflicts between 1 and 2 percent of the world's population. That translates to well over 2 million Americans and over 50 million worldwide. It is three times more common in women than in men. The onset becomes increasingly more common with age, peaking between the ages of thirty-five and fifty-five. People with RA may be burdened with three times the cost of medical care, twice the number of hospitalizations, and four times the number of physician visits. The lifetime cost to the person with RA may be as much as $250,000.

WHAT IS JUVENILE RHEUMATOID ARTHRITIS?

The term *juvenile rheumatoid arthritis* (JRA) may sound simply like RA which happens to develop in children, but it is actually a general label for three different forms of childhood arthritis that are quite distinct from the adult form. JRA develops more often in girls than in boys, usually during the toddler or early teenage years. JRA affects about thirty thousand to fifty thousand children in the United States.

Systemic onset JRA, also called *Still's disease*, affects many systems of the body. It often starts out as periodic fever and chills, which may go on for weeks, often accompanied by a rash on the thighs and chest. Along with a few inflamed joints, various bodily organs such as the spleen and liver may enlarge, and there may be inflammation of the liver and heart.

In contrast, *polyarticular JRA* may affect many joints including the hands, knees, ankles, feet, and hips. In some cases the protein known as the *rheumatoid factor* is found in the blood along with a genetic factor that is also common in adults with RA. Where the factor is lacking, the potential for severely damaged joints is less.

In *pauciarticular JRA* generally four or fewer joints are

inflamed in an asymmterical fashion; that is, if one knee or wrist is affected, the opposite isn't. There are various subtypes here as well, some of which may damage the eyes or the spine.

Many of the same medications now used for RA are given in JRA as well. The same kinds of fundamental research questions that are being asked about RA in research laboratories around the world are being asked about JRA. What sets off the immune system on the series of reactions that leads to and sustains these diseases? What are the interactions among the genes, the cells and perhaps even bacteria or viruses that spark and then fan the flames of these disease processes? Learning more about these interactions is to offer insights into new ways to diminish those flames and even perhaps extinguish them. While JRA and RA are different diseases, we may uncover crossroads where their paths meet in the biochemical reactions within our cells and tissues.

How Is RA Diagnosed?

Part of the diagnostic challenge is the fact that, as we've seen, there are a number of other forms of inflammatory arthritis that may share some similar symptoms. These include systemic lupus erythematosus (SLE), commonly known as lupus; ankylosing spondylitis; Reiter's syndrome; and the arthritis linked to psoriasis and colitis. While the emphasis of this book is on RA, it is important to realize that the search for ways to control RA at the cellular and molecular level will no doubt assist in the treatment of these and other often serious conditions as well.

There are several blood tests that may aid in the diagnosis of RA, but no one lab test will give a definitive answer. It would be ideal if the presence or levels of a unique, specific chemical in the blood—a *biochemical* marker—allowed a definitive diagnosis and could predict the progression of RA, but such a marker has yet to be found.

During the acute phase of marked pain and swelling the *erythrocyte sedimentation rate* (ESR), or "sed rate," test can be a useful indicator of the level of inflammation. This measures the rate at which the erythrocytes (red blood cells) settle out after being placed in a thin glass tube. The cells clump together and fall to the bottom more rapidly when certain proteins that are the result of inflammation form in the plasma, the liquid portion of the blood.

The blood levels of another biochemical, the *C-reactive protein* (CRP), made by the liver in response to inflammation, may be greatly elevated in early RA. Other blood analyses may reveal anemia, a decrease in the oxygen-carrying capacity of the blood, which is common in inflammatory diseases.

Between 75 and 85 percent of people with RA test positive for the presence of *rheumatoid factor*, an immune system protein that forms in the blood, usually before the end of the first year of the disease. The factor is made by certain types of white blood cells, the B cells, which will play a central role in the drama unfolding in the inflamed tissues. In this case these particular B cells seem preferentially to home in on the joints and gather there in great numbers.

To complicate matters, many people with RA can be *seronegative*, that is, they never develop the rheumatoid factor protein. Interestingly, between 1 and 5 percent of normal persons, as well as people with certain viral or bacterial infections or other rheumatic diseases, can have the rheumatoid factor in their blood. It is true, however, that people who persistently show high levels of rheumatoid factor within three years of the onset of the disease will develop the most severe symptoms. Whether or not this is a direct result of the presence of the factor is not yet known.

Sometimes the physician may withdraw fluid from a

swollen joint, such as the knee, in order to support a diagnosis of RA and to rule out other cases of joint swelling and arthritis. Microscopic examination of the sample for certain cells and chemical analysis can be very helpful.

So, various laboratory tests are useful to a degree for the purposes of both diagnosis and following the progress of RA. In the final analysis, however, the diagnosis is based on clinical grounds, that is, on the symptoms observed by an experienced physician.

RA can present many faces. It may begin abruptly or gradually. Sometimes events such as infections, injuries, surgery, or childbirth precede the onset of RA, but it is uncertain whether or not these can actually trigger the onset of the disease. The joints of the wrists, hands, and feet often are hit first, although stiffness and pain may strike first in the knees and ankles. A characteristic early complaint is joint stiffness upon awakening that sometimes lasts for hours. This is caused by an accumulation of fluid in the inflamed tissues during sleep. The swelling gradually subsides as the fluid is absorbed back into the blood when the joints start moving and flexing.

The affected joints are often swollen, warm, and tender, and may have limited motion. The "classic" RA is symmetrical, that is, typically both of the hands, knees, ankles, and feet are affected.

An accurate diagnosis takes time. One reason is that the full range of symptoms may not appear simultaneously. Another is that some of the symptoms of RA are shared by other forms of arthritis. Physicians typically use a set of diagnostic criteria established by the American College of Rheumatology (ACR; www.rheumatology.org),the professional organization of *rheumatologists* and associated health professionals dedicated to treating people with arthritis and other disorders of the bones, muscles, and joints.

A person is regarded as having RA if he or she satisfies *at least four* of the following seven criteria. These standards require that criteria one through four be present for at least six weeks:

- Morning stiffness in and around joints lasting at least one hour before maximal improvement
- Simultaneous swelling around at least three joint areas
- At least one joint area swollen as above in wrist, knuckle, or the middle joint of a finger
- Simultaneous involvement of the same joint areas on both sides of the body
- Nodules (lumps) under the skin
- Rheumatoid factor in the blood
- Radiographic (X-ray) evidence of erosions ("wearing away" of cartilage into bone) of hand or wrist joints

Note that the above criteria are used to precisely define RA for research. Ordinarily, if a person has only two or three of the criteria but also has erosions, for example, in the foot joints, this would still be considered RA. Although the above useful criteria do not include other signs, remember that RA is a *systemic* disease. It not only attacks joints, but can also result in mild fever, loss of appetite and weight, fatigue, or muscle weakness. Aggressive RA can produce relatively rare but sometimes serious complications. People with RA may often experience irritation of the cartilage in the vocal cords, resulting in laryngitis and in occasional trouble swallowing. In other cases the tear glands and ducts may become in-flamed, which leads to dryness in the eyes and mouth. Some-times this is actually *Sjogren's syndrome*, another autoimmune disease that can also affect other organs of the body including the kidneys, blood vessels, lungs, and liver. In rare cases the pericardium, the moist membrane around the heart, can become swollen and saturated with fluid, interfering with the normal heartbeat. In other uncommon expressions of RA, *vas-*

culitis may develop—large and small blood vessels become inflamed, which may result in skin ulcers, nerve numbness, or damage to internal organs.

What Happens to People with RA?

Here is a simple yet complicated question. If you and I receive a definite diagnosis of RA, what can we expect will happen to us over the months and years ahead? The objective, statistical facts are as follows.

In people with mild RA (between 5 and 20 percent), there is a spontaneous disappearance of symptoms, usually within the first two years. However, more than 50 percent of those will have a recurrence of RA with various levels of severity. Another 5 to 20 percent have a more progressive course, leading to some deformity of the joints. The majority of people with RA undergo a pattern of persistent and progressive deterioration that aggressively destroys cartilage and bone. More than 80 percent are partially disabled within twelve years after the diagnosis of the disease, and 16 percent are completely disabled. Median life expectancy is shortened an average of seven years for men and three years for women.

Given the statistics, you should remember that *the progression of RA often cannot be predicted in a given individual.* Predictions based on graphs, charts, and statistics yield only impersonal numbers. Persons with RA are individuals, each with a unique set of genes, health histories, and unmeasurable reserves of physical strengths and weaknesses that defy infallible prediction. At the same time we need to be realistic and admit that RA is usually a disease which now can be slowed down, but not stopped. We now know that prompt diagnosis and early, aggressive treatment can go a long way in modifying the advance of RA. This realization adds urgency to the efforts underway to understand RA and deal with it much more effectively.

WHAT ARE AUTOIMMUNE DISEASES?

Not only is RA within the category of arthritis, it is a charter member of one of the numerous *autoimmune diseases* that plague humanity. To have *immunity* to a particular disease is to be resistant to it. When you were vaccinated as a child, those quick and relatively painless injections resulted in one of the major achievements of twentieth-century medicine—your immune system was stimulated to protect you against diseases such as polio, diphtheria, whooping cough, and tetanus, which have attacked and often killed literally millions of humans.

We are accustomed to thinking about immunity as protection against invasions from microorganisms in the environment—bacteria, viruses, fungi, or protozoa. The complex and finely tuned immune system in our bodies consists of a varied array of cells and chemicals that recognize these creatures when they enter our tissues and that surround, attack, and destroy them before they can do serious harm. This defense system may not even need vaccinations to render us immune to some of the diseases caused by these microbes. For example, the first attack by chicken pox, measles, mumps virus, or even tuberculosis bacteria may be met by our immune system with a vigorous response, resulting in only minor symptoms and, from then on, permanent immunity.

In order to attack and neutralize the invaders, our immune system is equipped with detectors that can recognize them as outsiders to our bodies—as foreign; literally, creatures that are not us. In other words, we can distinguish what is "nonself" from "self," and set about to destroy the former. But all living cells, whether they are bacteria, muscle cells, or any other cell types, share many of the same kinds of molecules. We need to have a very efficient mechanism within the immune system to prevent it from mistakenly detecting our own cells as foreign invaders.

Occasionally, for reasons that we do not yet fully understand, that very mistake happens and we experience autoimmunity, an immune response directed toward self—toward one's own body. The results of this response manifest themselves as a wide variety of autoimmune diseases.

While autoimmune diseases have in common the unfortunate aspect of our immune defenses virtually biting the hand that feeds them, the more than eighty types of autoimmune diseases differ widely in their effects on the body. There are two major categories: organ-specific and non-organ-specific.

In organ-specific disease, the autoimmune attack is directed mostly at one organ. For example, pernicious anemia affects the stomach; Hashimoto's thyroiditis, the thyroid gland; Addison's disease, the adrenal gland; and insulin-dependent diabetes mellitus, the pancreas. Non-organ-specific diseases such as RA, SLE, and dermatomyositis have more widespread effects on many areas of the body.

Some of the diseases listed above may sound familiar; others may not. In fact, it turns out that the more than eighty known autoimmune diseases comprise the third major category of illness in the United States and many other countries as well, behind heart disease and cancer. One in five Americans has an autoimmune disease and almost 75 percent of those are women. The American Autoimmune Related Diseases Association, Inc. (www.aarda.org), is dedicated to the eradication of autoimmune diseases by supporting and integrating research on and education about this complex of diseases, which ranks as one of the world's major public health challenges.

So, What Causes RA?

One of the great mysteries associated with RA, or, for that matter, with any of the autoimmune diseases, is the vital question of what triggers and sustains the inflammatory eruption that can have such devastating long-term consequences. So far I have described only the effects of the disease. We know that it erupts within our immune systems. We can trace, to a degree, at least the course of the disease as it expresses itself in a variety of painful ways in different people.

At this point the general consensus is that there probably are a number of different factors that can set off this internal storm. As we have pointed out, the immune system normally can distinguish "self" from "nonself." To be a bit more precise, some of our *lymphocytes*, the type of white blood cells that are key players in that recognition process, have the potential to react against our own tissues, but are usually suppressed from doing that. In fact, those that do react in that way are usually destroyed before they can do harm. It appears that in RA there may be some interruption of that mechanism for control of "self-recognizing" lymphocytes. Also, there is evidence that there may be some alteration in certain body tissues so that they are no longer recognized as self and are interpreted as foreign invaders and attacked.

Exactly what causes this lack of control or tissue change is not yet known. There appears to be a mix of contributing factors: a genetic (inherited) predisposition, problems with white blood cell controls, and the presence of environmental factors including perhaps certain microbial infections, all of which might result in a bypassing of the normal processes of recognizing self.

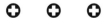

There are obviously vital questions remaining to be answered before we can more effectively control and even cure RA. However discouraging this may sound, remember that in science a clue to a single puzzle may lead quickly to its solution—as well as the solutions to other related questions. Scientists get at answers by "educated guessing," an accurate description of the more technical term of "developing a scientific hypothesis." A scientific hypothesis is simply a proposition, based on all the available knowledge, that is tested in as many ways as possible to either support it as correct or discard it as incorrect.

Regardless of how attractive a hypothesis might seem, it will never be useful unless there is sufficient proof of its validity. And what do we mean by proof? In science we mean evidence—facts—results that can be observed, measured, and reproduced. In the study of a disease this generally means experiments, observation, and analysis in the laboratory, followed by tests with experimental animals and, finally, with human volunteers.

In the search for the causes of RA and the precise details by which the immune system continues on a course of inflammation, cartilage loss, and bone erosion, there are numerous hypotheses that now are being tested and analyzed in ways not possible just a few years back. Evidence is being gathered in laboratories and clinics around the world as researchers examine the immune system step-by-step, constructing and testing hypotheses at each stage.

All of this is leading to evidence that supports the idea that there are multiple steps in the immune system that lead to the devastating effects of RA and the other autoimmune diseases. Scientists are using powerful tools of modern molecular biology to zero in on many of those steps to try to find a way to prevent our immune system from turning against us while maintaining its ability to protect us as it normally does.

Whereas it would certainly be satisfying and useful to

uncover all of the precise causes and mechanisms of the disease processes in RA, it is not necessary to wait until that happens before we develop ways to block their effects. There are now new medications, based on research, that have been approved for treatment (chapter 8) to supplement or replace some of the drugs that have been used for years for RA (chapter 7), while many other pharmaceuticals and novel approaches leading to treatments are under active development (chapter 10).

Our desire here is to trace the story of that search and provide a guide to understanding and following the progress being made to control rheumatoid arthritis. In order to do that we need first to go beyond the limits of unaided human vision and enter the microscopic world deep within our body's organs and tissues. We have to read the secret language of our cells.

CHAPTER 2

The Defenders

The extraordinary architecture of our bodies is based on one building block—the *cell*. Each cell is a microscopic living unit that aggregates with others of similar size and shape to form *tissues*—such as muscle, nerve, connective, or fat tissue. Various tissue types interweave and construct organs like the kidneys, pancreas, liver, or brain. Particular organs and related tissues fashion organ systems, including the reproductive, digestive, nervous, and immune systems.

The many trillions of cells that make up the human body are certainly widely diverse in form and function. For example, special cells which are shaped and arranged like parallel rows of dominoes line our small intestines and collectively offer an enormous surface area to the passing food particles. Vital food molecules are absorbed through these cells and pass into blood capillaries poised just beneath the epithelial layer.

The capillaries themselves are tiny tubes made of a single layer of flat, smooth, flexible cells through which dissolved materials can pass from the blood to the tissues and vice versa. The capillaries will permit the exit of white blood cells into the tissues under only unique conditions—such as inflammation. Our red blood cells are so small that 4 or 5 million are contained in a tiny droplet, and white blood cells are only a bit larger.

While cells assume many forms and have diverse functions such as contraction, secretion, or transmitting nerve impulses, they have in common the fact that each cell is a specific unit of living matter, wrapped in a delicate *cell membrane*. This vital wrapping, a complex of fats and proteins, determines what may enter and leave the cell. The cell membrane is, in essence, the gatekeeper.

What happens in a living cell? The answer is deceptively simple—its only activities are chemical reactions, otherwise known as *metabolism*. If one could perch on the cell membrane and watch cellular life in action, one would witness a dazzling array of thousands of rapid chemical interactions. But this would not be the chemistry of the test tube or the laboratory bench. This is the chemistry of life itself, a maelstrom of swirling molecules, seemingly random in their activity, but upon close examination strictly ordered—a tightly regulated dynamic chemical sea.

What drives these reactions? What makes them possible in the first place? Many of the chemical reactions are brought about by special *proteins* called *enzymes*. The critical importance of enzymes is their ability to assist molecules in combining with other molecules to form new combinations or to allow more complex molecules to break down into smaller components. The specific enzymes that are available to a cell are made under the direction of the cell's *genes*, which are located on the chromosomes. It is convenient to picture chromosomes as long strings of beads, with the genes being certain specific sequences of those beads. In any individual each cell has the same set of forty-six chromosomes (except for sperm and eggs, which have twenty-three). Inside the cell the chromosomes are actually long, densely tangled, threadlike molecules made of DNA and are located in the center of the cell within a special compartment, the nucleus.

Each set of human chromosomes contains all of the thirty to forty thousand or so genes (that number is as yet far from certain) that make each of us a human being, identical in many to ways to all humans but still, because of the particular combination of chromosomes inherited from our parents, a unique individual.

So our cells carry out their ceaseless round of chemical reactions under the direction of our genes. Genes make proteins, many of the proteins act as enzymes, and the resulting cell chemistry is what we call, collectively, life.

Proteins are central to life. Not only are they used as enzymes, they also form the structural framework for building cells and membranes and make up many of the molecules in the various crucial metabolic pathways in living cells, including much of the immune system. Proteins are able to carry out so many varied structural and functional roles because of the way they are put together. Twenty different building blocks, the *amino acids*, are strung together in chains hundreds or even thousands of amino acids in length in order to form *polypeptides*. These polypeptide chains, sometimes alone or combined with other such chains, are the proteins— chains twisted back upon themselves so that any particular protein is a complex coiled molecule with a specific sequence of amino acids. Given this potential for various shapes and structural sequences, there are many thousands of unique proteins, each of which has a specific role to play in living cells.

In any given cell at any one time most of the genes lie dormant, and only specific genes function, depending on the location and function of the cells in question. For example, cells near the surface of our skin are intent only on developing into flattened, waterproof protective layers, while the long tubular muscle cells in the biceps are busy making and maintaining interlocking protein filaments that glide over each other in opposite directions, resulting in strong, smooth muscular contractions. Genes in white blood cells, which are so important to our immune systems, are committed to making certain enzymes for manufacturing chemicals that help to guard against outside intruders like bacteria or viruses.

It certainly makes sense that all the genes in any one cell could not possibly function simultaneously. After all, each cell contains all the genes required to form and operate a complete human being. But what determines why some genes sleep while others work? As with almost everything that goes on in the human body, we do not know all the details of that regulatory process. We do know, however, that there are chemicals that are assigned to turn gene activity on or off depending on what is going on within the cell and in its environment, both nearby and far away.

Despite the fact that our bodies are made up of a far-flung empire of countless cells organized into tissues, organs, and organ systems, these parts cannot act completely independently of each other. Living cells need a constant supply of energy brought to them and a means of disposing of the chemical waste products of their metabolism. They must all somehow act in such a way that their activities are integrated and add up to a healthy (under ideal conditions), living, breathing, and moving human organism.

Our particular interest here is to take a close look at just one of the ways in which this extraordinary mass of cells called the human body maintains itself—not as a cluster of independent parts, but as a functioning community. We are interested in asking exactly how that community manages to protect itself from the constant barrage of outside invaders that threaten to attack, damage, or even destroy cells, tissues, organs, and, in some cases, the entire body.

Even more specifically, we want to introduce the basics of

what is now understood about how and why those powerful defense mechanisms, known as the *immune system*, sometimes turn their weapons against us in the form of rheumatoid arthritis. The more clearly medical science comes to understand how and why these painful events occur, the more hope there is of further success in devising ways to prevent them from happening.

THE IMMUNE SYSTEM

The human immune system is an intricate, dynamic drama of stimulus and response featuring a cast of thousands—or, more accurately, billions—of cells, a language understood only by the players, and a setting that includes every scene in the human body.

Cells are living sacs of chemicals. Cells neither feel nor hear nor see. They can know nothing about their immediate surroundings or, for that matter, what might be happening in other parts of the body beyond what arrives at their borders as chemical signals. The language that cells use is spelled out in molecules. Just as Morse code or, in a more modern context, electronic bits and bytes arriving at a computer are translated into meaningful parcels, the chemical messages that arrive at the cell borders are translated by the cell into commands that alter the cell's own chemistry in some way.

Cells detect these signals when the chemicals combine with specific *receptors* on the cell membrane, which then relay the information to the cell's interior. These receptors are special proteins, which can be thought of as padlocks; they will open up only in response to the right key. Depending on the chemical message that the unlocked padlock lets inside, the cell may respond by switching on or off specific genes or perhaps slowing down or accelerating their activity. Through this constant monitoring of the chemistry of its environment, a cell acts in a way in keeping with the messages brought to it from near and far.

The result? A living, active human individual whose trillions of cells, by responding to what they receive as chemical commands, react by adjusting their own chemistry. Despite the fact that one might reasonably perceive the human body as an impossibly chaotic system of interacting cells, most humans spend much of their lives in reasonably good health. That is, our body's chemistry in its totality operates in a comfortable equilibrium.

But as we all know, things can and do go wrong more often than we would prefer. We face two sets of dangers, one from within the body, the other from without. Within each cell the very genes inherited from our parents, the motors that drive the operations of our living cells, can include in their numbers defective members that can wreak havoc in the form of *genetic diseases*.

Those genes may express themselves directly as specific diseases such as cystic fibrosis, sickle-cell anemia, hemophilia, or Huntington's disease. Some of these genes have been identified, which provides us with knowledge to be used in diagnosis and in research aimed at treatment or even cure. But many of the body's disorders are linked to genes whose identities are not yet clearly defined and whose contribution to the problem is not yet completely characterized. Good examples are diabetes, cancer, Alzheimer's, and rheumatoid arthritis.

While these diseases have genetic components, only some of which have been identified, there are other contributing factors required for the expression of disorders such as RA. The search for the specific identities of those factors, such as injury, infection, diet, exposure to chemicals, or other signals, is an important part of the quest for ways to treat or cure literally thousands of diseases. In chapter 4 we will, with the goal of possible therapy in mind, look at the genetics of RA and consider what genetic predispositions might have a role in triggering the onset and influence the course of the disease.

What about attacks on the body from the external environment by invaders such as bacteria or viruses? Just as RA has an inherited, genetic side to its development, these invasions also are intimately connected with the story of how we develop RA. There is a school of thought (among others that we shall discuss) that maintains that RA begins with an attack by specific bacteria or viruses. Some of the protective responses of the body to the arrival of these dangerous organisms mirror some of the very same responses that the immune systems of people with RA make toward their own tissues. In the former case, bacteria and viruses are attacked and destroyed by cells and chemicals. In the latter, the same efficient weapons are turned against the tissues of the joints and elsewhere, and the destruction wrought brings pain and disability.

✪   ✪   ✪

It is easy to see how cells might be influenced by the chemical molecules released by nearby cells. But how are cells made aware of events in distant tissues? How does the sudden arrival of invaders in one area set off not only a localized response, but a broad signal to the rest of the body that help is needed?

The reactions of our immune systems, not surprisingly, require cell workers and chemical messages and also a means of carrying those messages throughout the body. For that purpose we use two quite distinct but interconnected anatomical networks, the blood circulatory system and the lymphatic system.

TWIN RIVERS OF LIFE

Living cells demand a constant supply of food and oxygen, and a means of disposing of the waste products of their chemical reactions, such as carbon dioxide and water. In the blood circulatory system, blood is propelled forcefully from the muscular heart and flows through a series of arteries of increasingly smaller diameter until it reaches the smallest vessels, the capillaries. Here, some of the liquid portion of the blood is forced out through the capillary walls to flow into the waiting tissues, bringing welcome dissolved oxygen and nutrients.

The cells, exposed to the thin layer of fluid bathing the tissues, absorb needed materials and expel their waste. Much of this tissue fluid then flows back into the capillaries, mingles with the blood, and returns through the veins to the heart. As blood moves through the lining of the lungs and intestines, oxygen and food is gathered. Wastes are removed as the blood passes through the kidneys, liver, and lungs.

However, not all of the tissue fluid recirculates through the blood capillaries. Instead, the remainder that does not enter the capillaries diffuses into the *lymphatic system*. This vital network begins as a mesh of microscopic tubes coursing through the tissues—a sluggish one-way stream that, collecting tributaries from throughout the body, converges into large, thin-walled vessels. These empty their contents into the blood in major veins within the chest that lead to the nearby heart.

The lymphatic system is much more than simply another route available for recirculating tissue fluid. It is the essential framework of the immune system—a critical resource for the recognition of danger and a supplier of the tools that defend us against that damage. Situated along the course of the lymphatic vessels are hundreds of *lymph nodes*, masses of organized lymphatic tissues, which act as filters through which the tissue fluid, now called *lymph*, trickles. Large aggregates of these nodes are located under the arms, in the groin, in the neck, and elsewhere (Fig.1). Several organs, including the spleen, the appendix, and the tonsils are masses of lymphoid tissues

These lymphatic filters are filled with cells that are waiting to detect the slightest hint of danger in the tissues. As discussed briefly in the preface, if invaders such as bacteria get beneath our epithelium they are met by hungry scavenging cells, such as the macrophages. These scavenging cells engulf the invaders and destroy them—and that is just the beginning of the story. Some of the macrophages, having eaten their meal, slip into nearby lymphatic vessels and are carried in the lymph stream to the nearest lymph node.

There the macrophages present specific fragments of the remains of the invaders to cells waiting in the node for just such a signal. These presented fragments are the *antigens*— specific pieces of the invader, usually proteins, that the immune system recognizes as dangerous. Alarmed by the prospect of an attack on the body, these waiting cells spring into action and set off a series of interdependent events that result not only in the production of protein *antibodies* specifically manufactured to combat the specific offending antigen, but also lead to the release of cells that join in the fray.

Antibodies are simply proteins that are able to grab onto matching antigens and see to it that the antigens are disposed of. If, as in the case of invading bacteria, those antigens happen to part of the bacterial cell itself, well, so much the worse for the bacterium. The antibodies mark it for destruction.

The newly recruited cell helpers leave the lymph nodes, flow through the lymphatic vessels to the blood and soon arrive at the affected tissues. There, powerful chemical signals persuade the cells to slow down, stop, and work their way through the capillary walls to join the ongoing struggle.

Because this scenario is so much a part of what goes on in RA, we must go beyond these generalities and look more

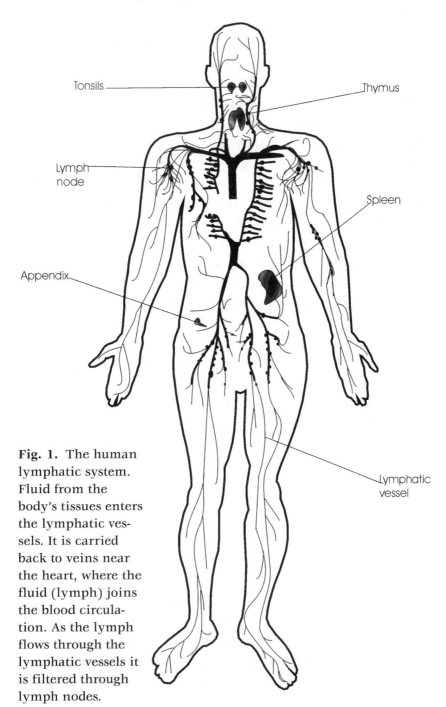

Fig. 1. The human lymphatic system. Fluid from the body's tissues enters the lymphatic vessels. It is carried back to veins near the heart, where the fluid (lymph) joins the blood circulation. As the lymph flows through the lymphatic vessels it is filtered through lymph nodes.

closely at the players in this immune system drama. While medical science does not have a complete grasp of all that goes on in this series of events, research throughout the world is intent on uncovering the details and using that understanding to devise more ways to intervene at each step.

The Players

In the human fetus the full skeleton is fashioned first as clear, flexible cartilage. Within the core of the longer developing bones, the *bone marrow*—a soft, rich tissue—begins to form from masses of cells called *stem cells,* which migrate there from the young liver. These stem cells have the capacity to differentiate into each of the six kinds of blood cells. Most will become red blood cells that carry oxygen from the lungs to the tissues. Others follow different paths and become *leukocytes*, the white blood cells designed specifically for the immune system. Some stem cells just make more stem cells, which remain in the bone marrow and continue to supply new populations of red and white cells throughout one's lifetime.

Of the various white blood cell types, the *lymphocytes* in particular need further preparation for their central roles in the immune system. This is crucial so that not only will the lymphocytes be prepared to recognize foreign invading antigens, they also must be conditioned not to mistake as dangerous any of the cells of the body, *the way they appear to do in RA*. In other words, they must be able to distinguish between self (any part of the body in which they are functioning) and nonself (anything else from outside that body). For example, the lymphocytes must be able to recognize and fight bacterial cells, but not recognize and harm cells from the person's muscles or joints. This vital learning goes on in several sites.

A portion of the newly minted bone marrow lymphocytes

are sent off from the bone marrow through the bloodstream like young students, to study in the *thymus gland* (Fig. 1). Before we understood the basic role of the thymus gland as a site of education for T cells, which is carried out in the early years of our lives, it was a most mysterious structure. That is because the thymus exists as a large, spongy mass in the upper portion of the chest cavity until the age of puberty at which time it begins gradually to shrink and almost disappear. We now know that this gland teaches the young lymphocyte to become a specific type of mature lymphocyte, the crucially important *T cell*.

Remember, cells communicate by means of chemicals. If all cells were sensitive to all of the chemical signals in their environment we would be in total chaos, much as we would be if our eyes and our bodies responded to every frequency of the spectrum, from X-rays to infrared light to radio waves. In short, we would have sensory overload. Just as our bodies have developed sense organs, like the ears and eyes, to pick up only some of those wavelengths, the T cells as well as other members of the immune system's cast of cells are sensitive only to very specific signals, that is, to specific antigens. They pick up these signals by means of protein *receptors* on their cell membranes.

The young T cells developing in the thymus gland in the chest will not survive unless they are exquisitely sensitive to nonself antigens, but simply ignore self antigens. In other words, they are not supposed to recognize any of the body's own chemicals, particularly the proteins, as "enemy" but should recognize chemicals from any outside source as such.

One of the extraordinary aspects of this recognition system is that individual T cells, and also *B lymphocytes* (*B cells*) as we shall see later, develop in such a way that each cell is capable of recognizing a different, specific antigen out of all the literally millions of antigens that a person might be exposed to during a lifetime. There are plenty of T cells to do this—we each have at least a trillion of them.

In addition to the *T cell receptors* (*TCRs*), most T cells also have *co-receptors,* which assist in recognizing antigens. It is as though it were not enough just to have a receptor that acted like a padlock, just waiting to be opened up by an antigen shaped like a matching key. The T cells use yet another lock that requires a different key. Primed with these receptors and co-receptors, the T cells are ready to sense and attach to antigens. The thymus now makes certain that these T cells will not react against self antigens. In other words, it must not allow the T cells to recognize the body's own tissues as dangerous and set off a damaging immune system response against them.

Within the thymus the T cells must pass a tough test. There the young T cells are exposed to samples of almost all of the antigens that the body carries—such as proteins from muscles, or kidneys, or cartilage. The way in which each T cell responds seals its fate. If it recognizes any self antigens, such as proteins from the body's cartilage or muscles as keys that open up its padlocks, the T cell will wither and die. This is the fate of at least 90 percent of the tested T cells.

The other T cells, which do not recognize self antigens, are allowed to leave the thymus and circulate in the blood for a few days, where they undergo some further selection to make sure that the T cells are healthy, functioning cells that are not harmful to self antigens. They then take up residence in the lymphatic tissues and recirculate between the lymph and the blood. In other words, our T cells are always on the lookout for the keys that will fit their padlocks and stimulate them into an immune system response.

Meanwhile, other lymphocytes in the bone marrow undergo maturation into B cells. Rather than head for education in the thymus, these young cells confine their studies to the marrow, where they divide repeatedly and come up with a dazzling variety of B cells. Each B cell becomes capable of making one specific type of *B cell receptor* (*BCR*), each of which matches one of the millions of antigens also recognized by the T cells. Each B cell is capable as well of synthesizing one of the millions of unique antibodies that match and lock on to specific antigens. In addition, the B cells can recognize many other antigens beyond those perceived by the T cells. As the B cells mature they are shuttled off to the lymphatic tissues throughout the body, where they take up residence near the T cells and circulate throughout the body, ever on the watch for signs of danger in the form of antigens.

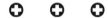

Now that we have introduced those cells that are active players in the immune system, we need to return once again to the drama that unfolds in response to an antigen attack and look more closely at some of the scenes that pertain directly to RA.

CHEMICAL CONVERSATIONS

The initial immune response is the one in which, as we out-lined earlier in a brief overview of inflammation, hungry cells called macrophages, waiting in the tissues, engulf the offending antigens, perhaps bacteria or viruses, and digest them. Physical damage to the tissues, as might occur in a wound such as a splinter or a laceration or when antigens are being ingested, causes cells to release a host of chemicals, including *histamine* and *prostaglandins*. You perhaps have taken *anti*histamines to give you relief from the symptoms of an allergy caused by antigens such as pollen or dust.

Soon, these chemicals expand the diameter of the local blood capillaries. Other powerful chemicals prod white blood cells to squeeze out through the capillary walls and then lure them toward the nearby site of inflammation Also, a specific type of white blood cell, the *natural killer cells (NK cells)* join the action, swarming in from the blood. They are specialists in killing tumor cells, virus-infected cells, and bacteria, parasites, and fungi. NK cells are three times as common in the blood of people with RA and twice as common in their joints, compared to the general population.

Meanwhile, a witches' brew of chemical messengers is being released by the feeding macrophages as well as other cells in the inflamed tissues. These are the *cytokines*. Certain cytokines play a central role in RA. At this point we will only make some relevant generalities about them and later come back to specific cytokines that are crucial to RA. The cytokines are a group of at least 150 different small proteins or glycoproteins (proteins with sugars attached), which include members that have effects that range from precise, local mechanisms to widespread general influences. A single kind of cytokine may be produced by a number of cell types and have numerous effects.

At least twenty-four different cytokines may play a role in RA. *Cytokines are the primary chemical messengers of the immune system—the language that the cells use to talk to each other.* The cytokines play a key role in developing and sustaining the early stages of the immune response, as well as that which follows later and fights the antigens with other weapons such as antibodies. We shall see in chapter 8 how some of the latest medications approved for RA act directly on certain cytokines.

Here in the body's first reaction to an attack, cytokines have wide-ranging effects. We now recognize that *rheumatoid arthritis includes a persistent, prolonged activation of the early immune system inflammatory response.* What might ordinarily have been a brief "mopping up" operation marked by a limited inflammatory period continues to the extent that the person with RA may experience a wide variety of harmful cytokine effects beyond joint damage throughout the body. These effects may include anemia, difficulty sleeping, skeletal muscle shrinkage and pain, and fatigue.

Meanwhile, after the early response, the immune response escalates. Urgent messages arise from the inflamed tissues where the initial reactions are taking place. The answers to those messages are both the manufacture of *antibodies* against the invading antigens as well as the activation of white blood cells that attack and destroy those antigens. Let's start with the B cells that make the antibodies.

B cells are born in the bone marrow. Amazingly, throughout our lives about one billion new B cells are produced each day. They each have many protein receptors on their surface, the B cell receptors, which recognize only one kind of antigen per B cell. These receptors and the antibodies are very similar in structure. Antibodies come in five forms all based on the most common one—*immunoglobulin G (IgG)*. The latter antibodies are literally Y-shaped molecules (Fig. 2).

Now in order for B cells to be activated into pumping out antibodies, several things must happen. First the B cell must somehow come in contact with the specific antigen that it can recognize among all others. This meeting may take place in the various tissues of the body or when the antigens trickle through the lymph nodes. The nodes are those lumps of lymphatic tissue that act as filters through which fluid returning from the tissues passes as it returns to the blood circulation (Fig.1). The waiting B cell receptors will grab onto the antigens to initiate the process of antibody formation. Often the antigen has already been recognized as dangerous and is covered with a coating of *complement*—a set of proteins that are always present in our tissues, ready to assist in our defense. So now we have B cells primed and ready for action against invading antigens. But they can't act quite yet.

Here is where the T cells come into the picture. They must physically interact with the B cells in a process known as *acti-*

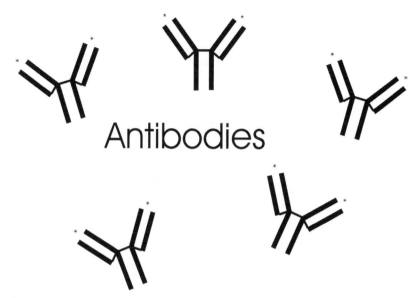

Fig. 2. Immunoglobulin G (IgG) antibodies. These Y-shaped protein molecules attach to specific antigens at the regions marked with asterisks.

---

vation, so that the B cells can finally make antibodies. But before they can be activators, the T cells also need some preparation; in fact, they themselves need to be activated.

Earlier in the thymus gland the T cells were decorated with molecules on their surfaces, the T cell receptors and co-receptors—those padlocks looking for unique antigen keys. There are specialized immune system cells designed to try the antigen keys in the T cell locks. They are called the *antigen presenting cells (APCs)*. These are either the hungry macrophages that have picked up antigens in the tissues, or B cells that have grabbed onto antigens, or a third category of APCs, the *dendritic cells*. The dendritic cells are abundant throughout the body. These flexible, starfish-shaped cells eagerly grab arriving antigens. Only these APCs bear the keys (antigens) that will unlock the padlocks on the T cells, and turn on the T cells to really get the immune system reactions going.

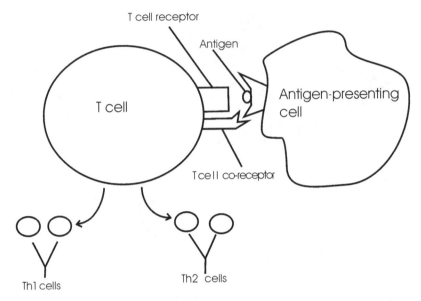

Fig. 3. Antigen-presenting cells, e.g. macrophages, can attach to T cells bearing the appropriate receptors and co-receptors. This will "activate" the T cells. The activated T cells then will divide into populations of Th1 (proinflammatory) and/or Th2 (anti-inflammatory) cells, depending on the presence of specific cytokine chemicals.

T cells that have particular types of co-receptors on their membranes, known as CD4 co-receptors, are the *T helper cells* (*Th cells*). The critical importance of these is underlined by the fact that HIV, the virus that causes AIDS, specifically seeks out and kills T cells bearing the CD4 co-receptors, in effect destroying the immune system.

So the T helper cells are major players in the immune system. In the lymph node, when T helper cells recognize and accept the antigen keys that are attached to the special antigen presenting cells described above, things really heat up. The activated T cells (influenced by certain cytokines) divide rapidly and build up a population of identical Th cells. After all, a single activated T cell won't be much help against an antigen attack. Now other cytokines come in contact with these

Th cells and the result is the formation of two distinct sets of Th cells, *Th1* and *Th2 cells*, each with different functions (Fig.3).

These Th1 cells and Th2 cells start pumping out their own unique sets of cytokine chemical messages. Meanwhile, other cells in the area are putting out cytokines as well. So the direction that the Th cells travel toward becoming either Th1 or Th2 cells is determined by the particular mix of cytokine messages sensed by the T cells. Once the choice has been made, the two Th cell types engage in different functions. *The Th1 cells are most interested in stimulating cells like macrophages and are therefore considered to be proinflammatory. In other words, in rheumatoid joints the balance seems to be swung toward Th1 cell activity, although Th2 cells are present as well.*

B cells are primed to make antibodies under the influence of Th2 cells. These activated B cells then have two choices. Some act as *plasma cells*. These cells churn out antibodies—about two thousand per second—and die off after a few days. The others become *memory cells*, which do not release antibodies but live much longer than the plasma cells. They or their descendants remain in the lymphatic tissues, acutely sensitive to the particular antigen that triggered this whole process. Should that antigen show up again in the body some of the memory cells will become plasma cells and mount a swift antibody response (Fig. 4). This is the basis of the immunizations we all receive as children. The injection of small amounts of antigens—measles, tetanus, hepatitis, and so on—initiates the manufacture and storage of waiting memory cells, which give long term protection against these once feared diseases.

Here we have yet another one of the many puzzles about RA. *Most (but not all!) people with RA have B cells that make antibodies that recognize some of the body's very own antibodies as foreign, that is, as antigens.* Whether or not these antiself antibodies, which we said earlier are called rheumatoid factor (RF), actually enhance the development of RA is not known.

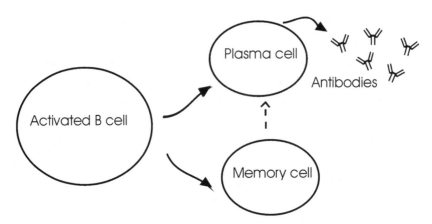

Fig. 4. B cells that have been "activated" divide into populations of plasma cells and memory cells. The plasma cells make antibodies. The memory cells, if the same antigen is present again, will quickly become plasma cells and make the appropriate antibodies.

There is some circumstantial evidence—RF is associated with the most severe expressions of the disease.

As you can see, our bodies are primed with a complex array of cells and chemicals prepared to repel any signs of danger. Most of us spend much of our lives in good health thanks to this silent whirlwind of activity going on within our cells and tissues. And yet it is also our human lot sometimes to fall victim to invasions that we cannot repel. For example, bacteria or viruses may enter our bodies and cause infectious diseases such as influenza, tuberculosis, pneumonia, or hepatitis, which may overwhelm the immune system's ability to cope.

In the case of rheumatoid arthritis, the immune system actually copes quite well in the sense that its working parts— B cells, T cells, antibodies, cytokines, and the like—go to work as they are programmed to do by their genes. *But now those immune reactions turn against the body's own tissues in answer to signals that we have not yet identified.* The search for those signals continues, as we shall see in later chapters. But already science is on the verge of understanding enough about the interplay between the cells and chemicals of the immune system during the painful progress of RA to fashion powerful new therapies to prevent pain, joint destruction, and physical impairment.

Let's look next at the sites from which much of this pain arises and where the cells and chemical messages that are summarized above interact so violently—the joints. In so doing we will also pinpoint precise steps in those reactions where some therapy for RA is already possible and where it will be more effectively directed in the future.

CHAPTER 3

Looking for Achilles' Heel(s)

From head to toe, each of our 206 bones connects to at least one of its neighboring bones at a *joint*. Some of those joints are simply slivers of dense tissue that bind together, for example, the flat interlocking bones in the skulls of young children. More flexible joints, such as where the ends of the two bones of the forearm meet, are formed by tough ligaments that bind the bones together yet allow some limited movement.

Our interest here is with the *synovial joints*, the most movable and most flexible joints in the body, which allow mobility in our wrists, fingers, shoulders, elbows, knees, ankles, and feet. *These are the joints that RA attacks*. The architecture of these joints is fitted perfectly to their functions. A tough *joint capsule* surrounds each joint and attaches to the edges of the bones like a loose-fitting sleeve. This assists the *ligaments*, which hold the bones together, along with the *tendons*, which attach muscles to the bones. This capsule of parallel, interlacing bundles of dense, white, fibrous tissue is richly supplied with nerves, blood vessels, and lymphatic vessels.

A delicate membrane, the *synovium*, forms the thin, smooth, moist inner lining of the joint capsule. It also extends out into *bursae* (sacs) near the joint that act as fluid-filled cushions between structures that would otherwise rub against each other, such as muscles or tendons. These bursae can sometimes become irritated and inflamed, resulting in the familiar pain of *bursitis*, a condition that may accompany RA but can occur as well in its absence.

Where the lower layer of the thin joint membrane, the synovium, merges with the fibrous capsule, the area is filled with blood vessels, fat cells, macrophages, and other cell types. The synovial surface consists of one or two layers of cells embedded in a firm, moist layer. Some of those cells can act like macrophages and when necessary ingest bacteria and debris within the joint. Other synovial cells secrete special chemicals that, together with fluid from the blood filtered through the membrane vessels, create a *synovial fluid* with the slick, gummy consistency of egg whites. *The first joint tissue to be affected by sustained inflammation is the synovial membrane. The inflammation spreads to the fibrous joint capsule and surrounding ligaments and tendons, causing more pain and stiffness.*

Using the knee as an example of a synovial joint (Fig. 5), note that the slender tibia bone of the lower leg meets the larger femur bone of the thigh. At this junction not only must the concave ends of the tibia support the weight of the body but they must also be able to glide smoothly beneath the convex protuberances of the femur as the knee flexes. The ends of the bones in flexible joints where bone meets bone are capped with pads of firm, slightly compressible living tissue, the *cartilage*, so that in these joints cartilage moves across cartilage, and the hard bony tissues never touch.

The synovium does not extend across the surface of this cartilage, but the synovial fluid does spread out across the cartilaginous pads, giving them a surface so slick that as the knee bends the two opposing cartilage surfaces glide over each other as smoothly as a well-lubricated hinge. The synovial

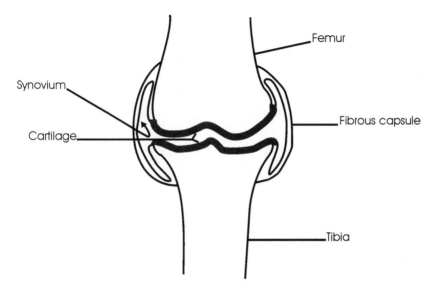

Fig. 5. The normal knee joint. Note that the ends of the bones are covered with smooth, protective cartilage.

fluid also soaks into the cartilage, supplying it with nourishment transferred from the blood.

The cartilage (Fig. 6) features live cells embedded in a clear substance rich with complexes of protein-based chemicals and strengthened with *collagen* protein fibers. When seen under a powerful microscope these fibers look like long steel cables arranged at various angles. At the cartilage surface they cluster tightly into dense, parallel bundles. Below, the fibers are more at an angle to the surface, allowing them to bend a bit and absorb some of the force of weight bearing.

The substance in which the fibers and cells are embedded is filled with large molecules of proteins, carbohydrates, and other chemicals. The carbohydrates include *chondroitin sulfate*. You might recognize this as a highly advertised nutritional supplement, along with *glucosamine*, for cartilage repair. There is little scientific evidence so far that these oral

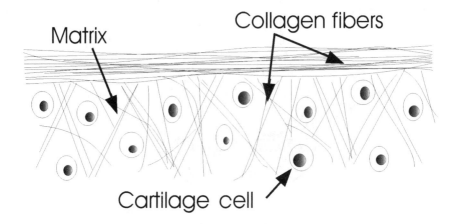

Fig. 6. The type of cartilage that covers the ends of the bones in the joints. The protein fibers and the cells are embedded in a dense "matrix," which has the consistency of rubber.

supplements are effective against RA, although extensive, carefully controlled research on this question was well underway in 2001. The natural chemicals within the cartilage are strengthening agents that help to regulate the slow movement of synovial fluid throughout the cartilage. Without these substances normal weight bearing would soon press all the fluid out of the knee cartilage. Certain of these molecules act as a kind of pump, allowing just enough fluid to be pressed out so that there is always a thin film creating a smooth, moist cartilage surface.

Motion and weight bearing are necessary to optimize this pumping action. In other words, use it or lose it. Prolonged nonuse of a joint reduces the effectiveness of this pumping mechanism and interferes with the nutrition of the living cells embedded in the cartilage. There are no blood vessels in the cartilage, so its health depends on the nourishment seeping into it from the synovial fluid.

HOW DOES RA START?

Biologists study a living system most effectively when they approach their subject with the assumption that given enough time, equipment, and perseverance, one can eventually learn all there is to know about it by understanding its building blocks, from muscles to molecules, and how these act in an integrated way. In a sense, they are seeking the "truth" about those complex operations summed up as "life."

But for any scientist the word "true" carries an element of danger. The danger lies in the temptation to accept as undeniable fact explanations that seem perfectly logical and have gained widespread support. Certainly there are many propositions in the world of science that have been proven to be accurate through careful observation and experimentation. Our red blood cells do carry oxygen in the blood, genes are certainly built from DNA, and we know that bacteria are all tiny creatures, visible only through powerful microscopes.

But wait—in 1999 biologists in Germany reported that they had discovered bacteria as large as the period at the end of this sentence, growing in ocean sediments. Why did this discovery surprise but not shock experienced biologists? Simply because they, like all scientists, must always leave the door open to accept further data. They always have to be open to the possibility of new evidence that what has been a comfortable generality, in this case about the size of bacteria, has been only a plausible story that can be disproved.

In other words, the only thing that impresses a scientist is evidence. That is why when we are trying to answer a puzzle we construct a *hypothesis*, that is, a seemingly logical explanation, and then proceed to try to put together evidence that will either support or contradict the hypothesis. Getting closer to home, the discovery that certain bacterial and viral infections often are found associated with RA has led to the suspicion, then hypothesis, that one or more of these microbes actually might cause the disease. It would certainly be good news if that were true, because then prevention by vaccine, which builds up protective antibodies, or cure of these infections with antibiotics, which attack the microbes directly, might lead to the prevention or cure of RA.

However, despite the appeal of this hypothesis, so far there is not enough hard-and-fast evidence to offer it as an acceptable answer to the question of what causes RA. If anyone wishes to defend this explanation as acceptable they have merely one requirement: offer evidence—data—that supports it.

Let's construct a scenario, bringing in several hypotheses, about the way that RA might begin that would involve microbes, though not necessarily directly. Assuming that RA is an autoimmune disease, it must occur because the immune system in an individual has failed to eliminate immune system cells that are "wired" to recognize that person's own cells as foreign, dangerous material (antigens). For this autoimmunity to develop further three conditions must be met.

First, the person must be able to make certain kinds of protein molecules that can present the self antigens on the surface of special antigen-presenting cells. Remember, the job of these presenting cells, such as the mobile macrophages always swarming about our tissues, is to take fragments of dangerous substances like bacteria and signal the immune system cells that danger is present. In this case, they unfortunately send the message that parts of our own cells are dangerous. That's the essence of an autoimmune disease.

This is one area where genetics comes into play. The genes that one inherits must be of the type that can make certain unique proteins on the surface of the antigen-presenting cells that hold out (present) the antigens.

Second, the person must be able to make T cells and B cells that have specialized receptors—sites on their membranes that will recognize those antigens. The millions of different subtle varieties of T cell and B cell receptors that develop as our white blood cells mature come from lots of different gene combinations. It is a matter of sheer chance whether or not this random receptor production will result in some of those white blood cells being able to recognize self antigens.

Third, it is apparently not enough just to have some T cells and B cells with receptors that recognize self antigens efficiently presented to them. There is more to it than that. *There must be other factors that lead to the breakdown of the normal tolerance mechanisms.* It is evident that autoimmune diseases sometimes follow certain bacterial or viral infections. However, most people who have these infections do not develop an autoimmune disease. One possible explanation (hypothesis) linking such an infection to, for example, RA is the concept of "mimicry." Here is how that might work.

It turns out that specific T cell and B cell receptors are not only capable of recognizing and locking on to one specific antigen fragment out of all possible fragments, but will have an attraction to one or a few pieces that are very similar. In other words, it is possible for them to "cross-react" with several antigens. This is what happens in mimicry. Certain bacterial or viral antigens might be picked up by scavenging cells, like the macrophages in our tissues, in the course of a microbial infection. Those antigens might be so closely related to certain self antigens that the alarmed T cells will cross-react with the self antigens. In other words, the T cells are fooled into confusing certain parts of the body with the invading bacteria or viruses. Following the instructions written in their genes, instead of just attacking the microbes to clear up the infection, they will start a campaign against the unfortunate person's antigens within their own tissues, thinking that they are microbes as well.

A classic case of such mimicry is rheumatic fever, so called because of the joint pain and fever associated with the condition. First, a particular form of *Streptococcus* bacteria causes a throat infection in a child. Antigens on these unique bacteria are so similar to antigens on the child's heart valves that the valves are attacked and damaged as though they were the invading bacteria, causing a serious rheumatic heart disease. The bacteria can be fought off with antibiotics, but the heart damage may be permanent, unless it can be corrected by surgery.

Now, in order to cause damage to us it is not enough for just a few cells to recognize a self antigen. These few cells that have reacted to the self antigen need stimulation by cytokines, those chemical messengers produced when the immune system is under siege, so that the few cells can multiply into millions. It appears that an inflammatory reaction probably must happen simultaneously in the person so that sufficient cytokines are available. With the help of a dose of those cytokines, these self-reactive cells can multiply and do damage.

For example, in RA there would have to be an infection in a joint by the "mimicking" microbe itself or perhaps another unrelated infection, or even an injury. In the resulting inflammation, antigen-presenting cells would pick up self antigens from the damaged tissues and present them to T cells able to recognize them, attach to them, and begin the process of further inflammation and damage.

Regarding RA, we know that it is a disease that affects the entire body and is characterized by persistent inflammation of the joints. The inflammation in RA appears to center around, among others, macrophages and the cytokine TNF-alpha, that powerful chemical that attracts immune system cells to the site of inflammation and helps activate them to fight against antigens. We do know as well that recent attempts to inactivate TNF-alpha in people with RA have resulted in some cases in measurable improvement (see chapters 8 and 10). In terms of mimicry there is evidence that T cells from some people with RA can "recognize" as antigens *collagen*, the major cartilage protein, as well as proteins of *Mycobacterium tuberculosis*, the bacterium that causes tuberculosis.

This *Mycobacterium* connection is interesting because the best-known example of inducing arthritis in animals (specifically rats) has been brought about through this bacterium. The specific factor in *Mycobacterium* noted in this reaction is a type of protein found in all cells, a so-called stress protein. One possibility, or hypothesis, is that these bacterial stress proteins could activate T cells in the joints, which would then cross-react with and attack similar molecules such as collagen in the joint cartilage.

Note that in this hypothetical sequence of events leading to the first stages of RA, even if the body were to kill off all the invading bacteria or viruses and leave no trace, the immune response would continue as though the microbes were still there because they are being mimicked by antigens in the person's own tissues. It's as though criminals had broken into your house and opened containers of toxic gas. Even if you could capture the trespassers, that wouldn't protect you from the poisonous fumes.

Other microbes as well have been suggested as possibly being linked to RA. These include the virus that causes infectious mononucleosis ("mono") and another virus associated with adult leukemia/lymphoma. However, the fact that traces of these viruses can be found in some people with RA is as yet only circumstantial evidence for their possible involvement.

Finally, our discussion of a possible connection between microbial infections and RA would not be complete without a reference to the ongoing studies on the role of bacteria called "mycoplasmas." The organism *Mycoplasma* is an unusual bacterium in that it lacks a cell wall and therefore takes on a variety of shapes depending on its environment. It is a very common cause of pneumonia. Since 1938, when Thomas McPherson Brown at the Rockefeller Institute first reported finding *Mycoplasma* in RA-inflamed tissues, the importance of this bacterium in RA has been disputed.

Only recently, in August 1999, the American College of Rheumatology reported the results of a four-year follow-up study of forty-six patients with RA who also had the rheumatoid factor in their blood. Their conclusions were that there was more relief from symptoms and less need for other medical therapies in some patients treated with the antibiotic minocycline. This is a form of *tetracycline*, the medication that for years has been advanced by followers of the late Dr. Brown as an effective RA treatment.

We'll deal further with this still controversial treatment in chapter 7. For now, note that this 1999 study did "not address the critically important question of the mechanisms of action of minocycline." In other words, this may prove to be not due to any antibiotic effect of the minocycline on the bacteria, but may have to do with the fact that minocycline may, among other effects, inhibit enzymes that are responsible for breaking down cartilage.

So, after all the above hypothesizing the question remains: Do, in fact, certain bacteria or viruses cause some cases of RA? To answer as a scientist one would have to say: We don't know yet. More evidence is needed. It is a fact that to date, no microbe has been found in joints or blood with sufficient regularity to furnish evidence to support this hypothesis. *As a matter of fact, using the same approach of hypothesis followed by experiments and observations, we can conclude only that there is not yet sufficient evidence to point to any specific factor as a cause of rheumatoid arthritis.*

The key phrase here is "not yet sufficient evidence." What this infers, fortunately, is that investigators are continuing to search for evidence for an agent or agents directly responsible for the onset of RA. However, as this search continues, *a new attitude is developing about RA as a "specific" disease.*

This attitude was neatly summed up by Rikard Holmdahl from Lund University, Lund, Sweden, in the April 2000 edition of the journal *Arthritis Research*. According to Holmdahl, "RA is probably not one disease, but, rather, a syndrome caused by several widely different . . . processes. In this respect, RA could be likened to a headache. No one would seriously think of trying to find a single explanation for a headache . . . it may be time to start thinking of a variety of different pathways leading to RA . . . it is time to accept that RA is a complex disease with multiple causes and pathways. . . . "

This attitude might strike one as discouraging in the sense that it seems at first to make RA even more complex than we might have previously thought. However, it is consistent with the approach of science. Holmdahl's comment, shared by many in the research community, is based on evidence. Within that body of evidence cited by Holmdahl are the many studies done in which various forms of arthritis are induced by a number of different means in experimental animals. The following is a startling example of how the complexity of RA has been revealed by such a study.

In 1999 scientists from Harvard Medical School working at the Institute of Genetics and Molecular Biology in Strasbourg, France, reported their analysis of blood taken from mice that develop a form of RA due to unknown causes. Healthy mice injected with this blood develop RA symptoms within just a few days. The researchers found that the substance initiating this reaction was a protein that is found not just in the joints, but in virtually every cell in normal mice—and throughout the normal human body as well.

What are the implications of this report? Does it just make things more complicated? Yes, in a way. But it is encouraging because it tells researchers that it may be productive, in the search for the causes and progression of RA, to look beyond substances found only in the joints.

⊕   ⊕   ⊕

Hypotheses relative to RA have to do not only with probing its origins but also the specific roles of the cells and chemicals that drive it along the path of inflammation and damage. Why? *Because given the fact that so far we cannot pin down a specific cause of RA and thereby prevent or cure it by striking at a known cause, or causes, we need to find out as much as possible about the pathways of inflammation and progression of RA within our joints and other tissues in order to know how to slow down or even halt those destructive events.*

To emphasize that important point, let's assume that we were interested in a problem completely unrelated to anything medical. Let's say that we were faced with having to set up an assembly line in a factory that could turn out hundreds of complete automobiles each day. In order to do that we would need to set up the sequence of workstations so that each part was put in place in the correct order. After all, if the axle was never connected to the wheels, the fact that everything else went smoothly would mean little—the car could not function.

Not only that, but each of the many parts that make up the cars would have to be ordered and placed at the correct place in the assembly line, ready to be picked up and added to the growing vehicle. Each worker would have to be trained to do his or her particular job—some might have to stay at one station, others would have to be more versatile. In the end, a complete car would roll off the line only if every step along the line had been carried out as planned.

Now picture the activities in a joint where RA has begun as a biological assembly line. What is being assembled there is a complex, full-fledged set of inflammatory reactions. That job needs a group of trained workers, in this case cells, such as T or B cells, or hungry macrophages. They are trained to do particular jobs by their genes. The tools that they use are not wrenches and drills but chemicals, and the cells have orders as to where and when they should use them. Of course, in contrast to the automobile assembly line, when all these cells and their chemicals are hard at work, following the instructions that have been handed down by their genes, what they build with great efficiency is used to just as efficiently dismantle something—the joint—and we feel the resulting pain, swelling, and loss of healthy function.

You have already read in chapter 2 about some of the (cell) workers and their (chemical) tools used by the immune system to assemble a beautifully functioning defense system. Now let's look again at that those same workers and their tools: workers forced by their genetic inheritance and some as yet unidentified commands to assemble a prolonged, destructive inflammatory attack against joints and other body tissues.

DESTRUCTIVE PATHWAYS OF RA

Let's examine the whirlwind of inflammatory activities in the joints of someone as RA develops, nevertheless remembering that *the precise progression of RA over time in different individuals may be similar, but it is not identical.* We will present this here in outline form only. Volumes have been and are being written in the scientific literature about these interrelated events. As an example, a computer search in late 2000 for technical information on the internal events in the development of RA yielded references to thirty-four hundred articles!

Our interest here is to look at the fundamentals of the RA inflammatory sequence as far as it is now understood, realizing that there is not yet universal agreement among scientists on every detail of that sequence. That lack of agreement, by the way, should not be discouraging. It is, in fact, a healthy sign. It means that every bit of scientific research on RA is held up to intense scrutiny by scientists, tested for accuracy, and compared with other findings to see if it contradicts or supports them. This is exactly how science makes careful progress.

Again, the following scenario is not meant to reflect an inevitable progression of RA in any one individual. The symptoms of RA vary widely among individuals. We are looking at a picture that represents the "typical" advance of RA in an individual who progresses to the severe stages of the disease. This is what may go on inside the individual's body as the months and years go by with RA.

⊕   ⊕   ⊕

As early symptoms of joint pain and stiffness appear, new capillaries form in the synovium (Fig. 5). The joint gradually swells with fluid seeping in from the blood. Hungry macrophages swarm actively and hold out antigens to T cells that have migrated into the joint. There has been some kind of injury to the joint tissues, perhaps from an infection, and lots of different antigens, including self antigens, are present. *Neutrophils*, white blood cells that pick up and destroy debris, similar to the actions of macrophages, accumulate in the joint fluid, now bolstered by added proteins and chemicals from synovial cells.

Certain sets of the person's genes, (some identified and others not yet pinned down), have instilled in that particular immune system the capacity to express a set of responses to these stimuli. Those responses, instead of simply resulting in healing of the initial damage to the tissues as might ordinarily happen in another person, set off an angry reaction within the joints that from then on can be slowed down by currently available treatments, but not stopped.

The T cells in rheumatoid joints are mainly of the T helper type 1 (Th1) category. These Th1 cells, (in contrast to Th2 cells, which slow down inflammation), promote inflammation by releasing stimulating cytokines. It's like the good cop, bad cop approach. Both can be useful, but sometimes, as in the case of RA, overdo it. (The importance of T cells in RA is underlined by the fact that individuals who contract AIDS experience almost complete remission of their arthritis—but at a very high price, of course).

Important chemical changes are underway in the small blood vessels in the area. Rather than move rapidly along in the bloodstream, lymphocytes (white blood cells) begin to slow down and roll along the vessel walls. There, sticky proteins on the wall, formed in response to chemicals seeping in from the nearby inflammation, latch on to attachment sites on the lymphocytes' outer membranes, as though two pieces of Velcro had met and stuck together.

This slows the lymphocytes. Once slowed almost to a halt, the lymphocytes adorn their surface with another protein. This in turn grabs onto a compatible protein on the vessel lining, stopping the lymphocyte. Quickly attracted toward the tug of chemicals oozing out from the inflammation, the flexible lymphocytes worm their way between the cells of the blood vessels and move into the inflamed synovium.

These lymphocytes include many neutrophils, which make up 70 percent of our circulating white blood cells. They must be important—about 100 billion neutrophils are made in our bone marrow each day, prepared to leave blood vessels and spend their alloted life span of only a few days wherever they are needed to pick up and digest invading microbes or whatever cellular debris needs disposal. In RA the neutrophils leave the blood vessels, move through the synovium, and enter the synovial fluid lubricating the joint.

There the neutrophils contribute significantly to the inflammation itself, as if firefighters were dropping matches at a blaze. In the chemical environment of the RA joint they leak corrosive enzymes and other chemicals, which attack the outer surface of the cartilage. At the same time some of those enzymes begin to degrade the molecules within the cartilage, causing the cartilage to absorb water and swell, leaving the cartilage vulnerable to mechanical damage from compression during weight bearing.

As these changes continue for a few months, T cells and macrophages emit cytokines, which provoke the synovial cells to multiply and increase the weight and volume of the synovium twenty to one hundred times its normal size. The majority of the cells in the swollen synovium are macrophages. These play a pivotal role in perpetuating inflammation in RA because they release (among others) the cytokines *tumor necrosis factor-alpha* (*TNF-alpha*) and *interleukin-1* (*IL-1*). *It would be difficult to overemphasize the role of TNF-alpha in RA. It plays a central role in inflammation and, as we shall see in chapters 8 and 10, it is a main target in the newest RA therapies.*

Meanwhile, B cells become active and make antibodies, including the rheumatoid factor—that antibody found in the majority of people with RA. One result of this is that these antibodies combine with antigens. These antigen-antibody complexes become covered with a layer of complement, those abundant immune system proteins. These interactions form *immune complexes*—clumps of sticky proteins that form deposits within the joint. These immune complexes attract and activate white blood cells, thereby propagating the inflammation even more. In later stages of RA, immune complexes may cause *vasculitis*—inflammatory damage to the lining of blood vessels.

Deposits of these immune complexes within the outer layer of the cartilage attract the attention of an invasive, erosive mass of tissue known as the *pannus*, a tumorlike tissue (Fig. 7) now forming in the synovium. Within a few months of the development of RA symptoms, the lining of the inflamed

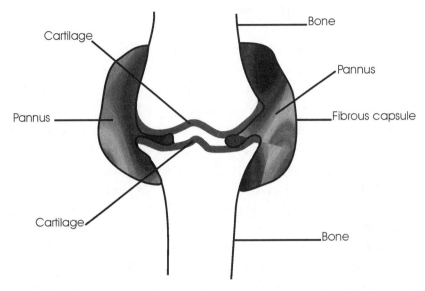

Cartilage

Bone

Pannus

Pannus

Fibrous capsule

Cartilage

Bone

Fig. 7. An inflamed joint, as seen in RA. Note that the synovial membrane has enlarged into a pannus, which can invade and destroy cartilage and bone.

synovium increases in depth and in numbers of cells, and becomes highly folded, extending into fingerlike projections that form the pannus. Elongated cells in the synovium transform under the influence of cytokines into aggressive dividing cells that release several kinds of cartilage-destroying enzymes. The pannus becomes a tumorlike tissue, slowly moving in from the edges of the joint toward its center, gradually eroding cartilage and even the underlying bones.

Within the masses of cells multiplying in the joint, some appear to have been liberated from the controlling signals that normally would have caused them to die. In the course of normal tissue development certain unneeded cells are neatly disposed of in a natural process. In RA there is evidence that some defects occur in this process of programmed cell death, which leads to a kind of abnormal stockpiling of cells in the joint.

During this progression from the early excitation of the immune system to the abnormal destruction of otherwise healthy tissue, many chemical signals are transferred among the cells taking part in the damaging process. I have mentioned only a few because they are among the best known chemicals, such as TNF-alpha and IL-1. However, there are numerous chemical conversations going on using at least ten other IL-type messengers. The latter are signals for communication between leukocytes (white blood cells), so they are abbreviated IL for "interleukins," that is, "between leukocytes." There are other categories of chemicals as well that keep fueling various aspects of the inflammation.

Prominent among those other chemicals are the *prostaglandins*. These are made by neutrophils, macrophages, and other cells in the joint in response to TNF-alpha and IL-1. The prostaglandins cause pain and also help to increase the flood of cells and fluid into the aching joints.

After several years of the disease, the person with severe RA loses mobility, and muscles shrink due to disuse because of pain. As the years pass, even more bone as well as surrounding tissues may be destroyed, leading to deformity of the joints and loss of function.

The cellular workers, using their elaborate set of chemical tools, have done the job assigned to them by their genes. In another (fortunate) person the same set of stimuli—perhaps infection and/or injury—would use many of the same workers and chemicals to fight off the intrusion, and heal the injury. The whole process would perhaps be little noticed. In a person prone to RA those seemingly innocent beginnings would turn the cells and their chemical tools toward their pernicious enterprise.

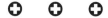

In trying to decipher exactly what goes on in RA at the level of cells and chemicals it is important to underline *that the disease occurs in individuals whose immune systems are generally competent.* Those of us with RA do not necessarily catch more colds, or suffer from more infections or allergies. In other words, as J. H. S. Gaston, professor of rheumatology at the University of Cambridge School of Medicine, so eloquently explains, ". . . [in rheumatoid arthritis the] immune system has some minor character defect that, as in all Greek tragedies, leads ultimately to disaster."

What is this "minor defect," (or perhaps there are several) that leads to RA? Until this can be more clearly defined, and I am confident that it will be, the logical approach is to gain control over as many as possible of the steps as outlined above along the assembly line of inflammation and destruction.

GAINING CONTROL

During RA and in many other autoimmune diseases, our immune system, while attacking and harming various parts of our bodies, nevertheless continues to protect us from other kinds of potentially damaging or lethal threats. Because those contradictory activities are simultaneous, it stands to reason that we cannot simply shut down a person's immune system in order to alleviate the damage and pain due to an ongoing disease. After all, the virus that causes the tragic disease AIDS does just that. Entering the T cells, it destroys them from within and as a result, effectively destroys the immune system. The T cells, as we have seen, are central to the immune system functions, stimulating B cells, for example, to make antibodies in order to fight infection. People with AIDS do not succumb to the virus directly but to what otherwise might be minor infections, now unchecked because so many of the T cells have been eliminated.

To use another example, successful organ transplants are only possible if the immune system reactions of the recipient are lessened. As far as the recipient's immune system cells are concerned, the transplanted organ, however closely compatible, is a large mass of foreign antigens and ought to be torn apart and removed. The person must be given powerful medications to suppress this natural defense, a regime which exposes that individual to greater risk of infection.

There is room for this dramatic approach in some situations with RA, as we shall see in chapter 6, but the ideal approach must be much more sophisticated. What we need to do is to gain control over the production and activity of the cells and chemicals at various points along the assembly line of RA. Because so many different cell types and chemicals contribute to the development of the disease, and because their functions so often depend on each other, interfering with just one step might not be enough to stop it.

We may need to block several steps along the way and as early in the progression of the disease as possible. At the same time we have to balance the effects of removing essential cells and chemicals from the assembly line of duty. Furthermore, if we do all this with medications, we have to balance the relief that they bring with the problems that the drugs' side effects might elicit. The ideal? A single therapeutic agent that will block most, if not all, the main stages along the assembly line.

Our insights into the inner workings of the immune system in health and disease have expanded enormously over the last decade and continue to clarify our still somewhat cloudy view of the complexities of RA. What are the most logical and possibly fruitful approaches that science and medicine can take to gain control over this disease? The following is a list of those approaches—not necessarily in their order of importance because any one of them might prove to be the most effective, a combination of several might emerge as a powerful therapy — or another as yet unforeseen method might trump them all.

- RA, in order to attract and import cells that create havoc, particularly white blood cells, to the scene of inflammation, needs new blood vessels in the tissues lining the joints. This sprouting of new vessels, known as *angiogenesis*, can now be inhibited as an experimental means of shutting off blood supplies to cancerous tumors. On the other hand, researchers are now attempting to stimulate angiogenesis in tissues where new vessels may be beneficial, such as in damaged heart muscle. In RA diminished angiogenesis would be desirable to close down vital supply lines bringing in harmful cells to the joints.
- B cells, because they make certain antibodies that attack joints and tissues in RA, might be somehow removed or destroyed, in hopes that the new population of B cells that the immune system would make to replace the troublemakers would not make these destructive antibodies.
- Chemical messages come from the tissues where RA is beginning and move to the local blood vessels. There, those chemicals help to fashion proteins along the vessel lining as well as proteins on the outer membranes of the white blood cells that stream by. All this helps the cells exit to carry on inflammation. These chemical messages cause the vessels to become "leaky" and the cells to slow down, lock on to the vessel lining, and then move quickly through the wall into the nearby tissues. Interference with those messages could prevent those cellular reinforcements from answering the call for help.
- The hungry macrophages, some of which are already in the tissues and the many others that are recruited from the blood, are central players in RA. They excite T cells, they pour out inflammatory chemicals (cytokines), and

even assist in cartilage and bone destruction. Anything that could reduce their numbers or their activity would be very useful.

- T cells are in the mainstream of immune system reactions. They recognize substances (antigens) presented to them by specialized cells such as macrophages. The T cells become "activated" and go on to perpetuate inflammation and damage to the joints. The T cells communicate with other cells by literal physical contact with them. They recognize other compatible cells, as should be no surprise by now, by sensing specific chemicals on the cell surfaces. Why not block those chemical identifiers, or plug up the sensors on the T cells? That would prevent interaction of the T cells with other cells and block the damaging aftereffects of those meetings. Because certain types of T cells, the Th1 cells, predominate in RA, suppression of their numbers and an increase of the antinflammatory Th2 types might help.

- Each of the cytokines, those chemical messengers that literally run the operations of the immune system reactions, are prime targets. Central among them, at least as we now understand it, are TNF-alpha and IL-1. These two have a hand in so many of the operations of immunity that some control over either one could be a very powerful weapon against RA.

- *Apoptosis*, the process that the body uses to carefully delete unneeded cells, seems to be defective in RA. It would be useful to stimulate apoptosis to get rid of particular cell types that are perpetuating destructive inflammation.

- In the destruction of cartilage and bone, powerful enzymes that dissolve those precious tissues are secreted by cells that have been excited by cytokines. A way to reduce or eliminate that flood of corrosive chemicals would reduce or prevent the painful damage.

- While we wait for a way to cure RA we certainly need to come up with new and better medications to suppress the pain that goes with it, for example, even more effective methods to suppress those nasty prostaglandin chemicals that induce pain.
- Perhaps a way might be found to vaccinate someone and make him or her immune to RA in the way we now protect ourselves against polio, measles, tetanus, and other diseases.
- Maybe we can we learn enough about the inheritance of the tendency to develop RA to predict where it will strike and then take preventive action. As we learn more about the genes that are responsible for the onset and the progress of RA, we might be able to learn how to adjust those genes in some way using the powerful tool of gene therapy.

These categories of possible avenues to the prevention, treatment, or cure of RA do not constitute merely a wish list. As a matter of fact, scientists in universities, medical centers, and biotechnology companies around the world are already making progress, to varying degrees, in every one of these approaches. Even as they uncover new details about the intricate relationships among the immune system cells and their chemical messengers in health and in disease, they are applying that new knowledge to develop specific therapies.

These therapies aim at striking RA where it is the most vulnerable—the pathways along that assembly line of smoldering inflammation and destruction. Several of these new therapies are available now while some wait in the wings for approval by the FDA (see chapter 10). Others are now at some stage of development from the laboratory bench to actual clinical trials. This revolutionary change in RA treatment will undoubtedly continue to expand throughout the early years of the twenty-first century. Let's now take a closer look at what we expect will be the near future of RA therapy.

CHAPTER 4

The Gene Hunt

Effective therapy for any disease depends on an understanding of the way in which the disease interrupts normal, healthy chemical processes going on within a person's cells and tissues. That knowledge, gleaned from careful observation and research, can be used to develop ways to intervene in the progress of that disease by interfering with its destructive tools.

Many illnesses caused by bacterial infections such as strep throat or abscesses, or fungal infestations such as athlete's foot, can be treated with antibiotics that kill the invading organisms and cure the problem. Viral diseases like polio, measles, or mumps cannot be treated with antibiotics, but the understanding of how to grow and manipulate viruses in the laboratory has led to vaccines that protect us from those and other viral parasites. As another example, we discovered that the insulin-producing cells in people with diabetes were damaged and that through insulin injections their lives could be saved.

Fortunately, intervention against some diseases may be so effective that the person is cured or even protected from future assaults. Often, however, while the treatment can give some relief from pain and other symptoms, it does not strike at the vital step(s) of a particular mechanism that the disease uses to disturb or destroy normal cellular chemistry. There are, for example, bacteria that are resistant to all antibiotics. There are viruses such as HIV, the cause of AIDS, for which no effective vaccine has yet been developed. And insulin, while it saves many lives, will not repair the damage to the insulin-producing cells of a person with diabetes.

Our interest here is in the possibilities for treatment, prevention, and even cure of RA. All of those possibilities, from more effective pain relief to complete cure, might perhaps be realized if the search begins deep inside the cells of a person with RA. We have to penetrate the membrane that separates the cell interior from the its surroundings; move through the cytoplasm, that viscous mix of interacting chemicals; pierce another protective membrane; and enter the nucleus, the master control center of the cell.

There, contained within the tightly coiled chromosomes of every individual, is the *human genome*—all of the genes of that person—the full set of instructions for making a specific human organism. It is the master program for building all of the body's structures and for carrying out all of its cellular chemical activities. That same genome resides in the nucleus of every one of that person's cells. The chromosomes in a nucleus are in two sets of twenty-three—one set donated by each parent. Each chromosome is one long, narrow, coiled *DNA* molecule, wrapped around clusters of protein.

Each of the thirty to forty thousand or so of the genes (that number is still just an educated guess) that make up a person's genome is a short segment within the DNA. A single DNA molecule, extending the length of the entire chromosome, is made up of hundreds of thousands of chemical building blocks called bases, linked side-by-side in one continuous chain. DNA is actually a two-sided molecule, shaped like a twisted ladder held together by rungs. There are only four different bases used in making DNA. They are referred to by the symbols A,

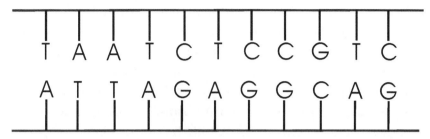

Fig. 8. This "ladder" represents a small section of DNA. The letters represent the four different types of bases, the building blocks of the genes. The difference between each of the thirty to forty thousand or so human genes has to do with the specific sequence of those bases. A typical gene might be between ten and twenty thousand bases long.

T, G, and C. The bases occur in pairs—either A with T or G with C—joined together across the "rungs." The long sequences of bases that make up the genes are located on one or the other side of the "ladder" (Fig. 8).

Very simply, what makes one DNA molecule different from another is in the sequence in which the bases appear in that DNA—for example A, C, T, A, G, C, A, and so on. An average gene would be a piece of DNA between one thousand and fifteen hundred bases in length. In the human genome there are approximately 3 billion bases, so the possibilities for variation in sequence between one gene and another are enormous.

The exact sequence of the bases, the building blocks that make up those genes within our DNA, while very similar among all humans, is not shared by any two people (except identical twins). We all share a common genetic inheritance that makes us a member of the human species, and we all share many of the same genes and gene sequences—yet we each have specific sequences in our DNA that make us unique—in health and sometimes in disease. (By the way, the genome of the corn plant has about 5 billion bases—it's the sequence that counts!)

The genes are arranged one after the other along the chromosomal DNA strands like beads in a chain, though often separated by intervening stretches of bases. Actually, about 97 percent of the DNA in the chromosomes is not part of genes. There are long stretches of base sequences between many of our genes—sequences whose functions are, for the most part, still a puzzle. Imagine that you are looking at a printout of the base sequence of an entire chromosome, searching for those bits of sequence that are genes. If the genes were words that you could understand, as you perused thousands of pages of random letters, you would occasionally come across a recognizable word. We do know for sure that each gene is essentially a code for making a specific protein. Here is where the importance of the base sequences of the genes come into the picture.

The simple principle here is that the sequence of bases in the DNA of each gene determines the sequence of the building blocks of the protein that they are in charge of making. Proteins are long chains of *amino acid* building blocks, often thousands of amino acids long. Cells have twenty different amino acids with which to construct proteins, so the possibilities for variation in protein sequences is enormous. Since the way the proteins function depends on their amino acid sequence, the instructions from the DNA are critical (Fig. 9).

In other words, in all creatures, from bacteria to humans, the same system operates to produce and maintain those complex structures and reactions we call life. Our particular genes determine the proteins that we can make—which determines our physical and chemical capabilities. You may want red hair, but no act of the will can make that happen *naturally*. You require the genes that will make red pigment—as well as the genes that will make the hair itself.

It is important to keep in mind, as we deal with genes that relate to RA, that while genes are in a real sense in charge of what we are and what we can do, those thirty or forty thousand or so genes in every human genome themselves are controlled by chemical signals. At any one time, only relatively few genes

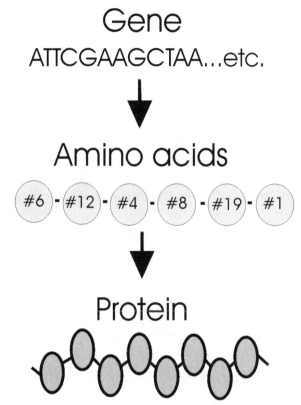

Fig. 9. A gene functions as a code for the manufacture of a protein. The sequence of bases in a gene determines the sequence of amino acids, the building blocks of the proteins. In this way, the genes determine the characteristics and activities of cells.

are making proteins, or as biologists put it, are "turned on." For example, in the cells of the retina of the eye and the muscles in the arm, there are exactly the same kind and number of chromosomes and genes. Obviously, not all the genes in these different tissues are turned on at the same moment. If they were, chaos would result. *An extraordinarily important area of research, certainly applicable to RA, is the identification of the control systems for regulating genes. In chapter 5 we will discuss specific examples of how some of these controls are already being put to the test for attacking RA.*

GENES AND RA

Many of the proteins made under the direction of the genes are critical structural components of cells and tissues such as cartilage and bone, and many other proteins act as enzymes, driving each cell's chemical reactions. It stands to reason, therefore, that the genes that we inherit from our parents are crucial to our state of health.

There are well-known diseases that can be attributed to a different single gene defect. The most common of these is cystic fibrosis, in which two copies of a faulty gene on chromosome pair 7, one copy from each parent, result in thick mucus secretions in the lungs and intestines. In Huntington's disease a single abnormal gene on chromosome 4, inherited from either parent, results in a progressive and fatal loss of muscular and mental functions, usually in one's adult years. These and several hundred other disorders depend simply on the presence of specific genes that one inherits in the genetic lottery of human reproduction. It is intriguing that only one gene out of each person's many thousands of genes could wreak such havoc on a person's life.

What do we know about the genetics of RA? Can it be inherited and therefore be passed on to our children? Is there any way to tell if we have "RA genes"? Can learning about the role of genes in RA help us in diagnosis and especially in treatment?

There are still many unanswered questions about the contributions of genes to the inheritance, onset, progression, and severity of RA. However, it is increasingly clear that RA is a disease that arises from a blend of multiple genes that contribute to a person's susceptibility, or risk, and which require for their operation other "triggering" events (also not yet clearly defined) such as infection or injury. That means that RA is not like cystic fibrosis or Huntington's, in which the presence of particular genes leads invariably to the disease.

Instead, there are genes that seem to be required to predispose a person to RA, without making it inevitable. Let's look first at the important question of the inheritability of RA.

We have known since the late 1970s that RA definitely has a genetic component. In order to determine its extent, researchers have compared the prevalence of RA among different groups of individuals with different degrees of genetic relatedness—genetically identical individuals (identical twins), fraternal twins and siblings, and unrelated individuals. The numbers change as more studies are done, but one can approximate that in the general population the chances of developing RA is 1 percent, while it is 2–4 percent for people with a sibling who has RA, and 12–15 percent for a person whose identical twin has the disease. Since identical twins both have the same genome, the disease is clearly not inevitable.

In other words, because there are genes that contribute to RA, the chances of having those genes is greater among people who are related, since they inherit many of their genes from the same pool of people. *In practical terms, if you have RA, the chances that your child will develop RA are somewhat greater, but the probability is so low that your RA is not considered a strong risk factor for your child. In short, it is not inevitable.*

But what are the specific genes that contribute to RA? And why is it important to track them down, the way we have identified the chromosomal location of many other disease-related genes? To answer the latter question first, the most compelling reason why we need to pinpoint the genes that contribute to RA is that in doing so we will have a means of achieving a better understanding of the disease process and be able to develop better therapies based on a clearer picture of the mechanisms of the disease. For example, specific genes crucial to RA could be used as targets for procedures that could block the effects of those genes. It might also be possible to identify the people who are at greater risk for having RA and use aggressive therapies to stop the disease in its earliest stages.

RA is a disease of sustained inflammation and tissue damage in which T cells, those abundant white blood cells, appear to play a central role. T cells are "activated" by detecting antigens, substances that the body considers foreign and dangerous to it. Those activated T cells, now referred to as helper T cells, release chemicals (cytokines) that perpetuate inflammation and destruction in a variety of ways. We do not yet know what particular antigens activate T cells during RA, but we do know something about the genetics of that crucial step.

The capacity that T cells have for antigen recognition is governed by certain genes. Those genes are located on chromosome 6, in a gene cluster designated as the *MHC* complex, usually referred to in humans as the *HLA*, the "human leukocyte antigen" system. This indicates simply that the HLA genes are in charge of making proteins that are used to act as "holders" that present antigens to those special white blood cells, the T cells, for their inspection. It is as though the cells such as macrophages, which the body uses to show antigens to T cells, need "hands" attached to their outer membrane in order to hold out the antigens for display. Those "hands" are proteins made under the orders of the HLA genes. This is done in two ways.

First, all cells of the human body "display" on their outer membranes fragments of the proteins that they manufacture, as though they were draping themselves with samples of all of their wares. One reason for doing that is so the T cells can periodically check other cells to be sure that they are not having problems, such as a viral infection. If certain T cell types detect viral proteins displayed on a cell they will quickly destroy the cell to prevent spread of the virus.

There are subtle but important differences among the genes in the HLA clusters of humans. This means that cells, tissues, or organs from one person (unless that person is an identical twin) will be recognized as foreign and dangerous if they are put into another person, as occurs in an organ transplant. The transplanted material will be attacked and destroyed unless powerful drugs are used to shut down that response.

Our concern here is with the other kind of antigen-presenting proteins that the HLA makes. These proteins are found only in the immune system. They are located on the outer membranes of those cells, such as the macrophages mentioned above, whose job is to pick up and present antigens that have entered the tissues from the outside—such as bacteria. Those antigen presenters—such as macrophages—actually ingest and kill the bacteria. They then select pieces of the bacteria—the antigens—and move them out to their cell membrane surface. As noted earlier, there they mount the antigens on their "hands," protein holders made under the direction of the HLA genes. These antigens, along with the protein holders grasping the antigens, form complexes that are recognized by special receptors on the T cells. They pay no attention to empty "hands." (Fig. 10).

This is an efficient, lifesaving system that operates in us around the clock, enabling T cells to recognize and respond to attacks of bacteria, fungi, viruses, even parasites. Unfortunately, in people with RA, a certain combination of HLA system genes may predispose them to activate T cells that recognize some of the person's own tissues as antigens and help to destroy those tissues, including cartilage and bone.

Within the cluster of genes that make up the HLA system, there is a region designated as HLA-DR which has long been recognized as somehow associated with RA. Each of the genes in this cluster vary slightly from one person to another, so that the proteins they make also vary. Studies of these differences reveal interesting comparisons among ethnic groups. For example, the so-called HLA-DR4 gene is found in 70 percent of

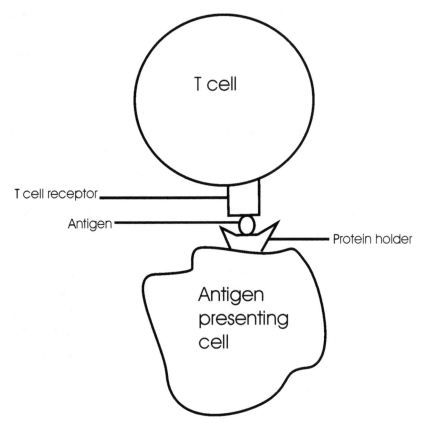

Fig. 10. The cells that present antigens to the T cells (see Fig. 3) do so by attaching the antigen to a special protein holder. In this way the T cell can recognize the antigen.

Caucasians with RA in North America. However, among African Americans with RA the incidence of this gene form is only 14 percent.

Genetic analyses looking for HLA genes that are linked to the genomes of people with RA have been carried out in many ethnic groups. In spite of the fact that it now seems clear that susceptibility to RA is not always associated with the same specific HLA genes in all people, there is a major hypothesis that has come out of these studies. *Many people who have RA have the same specific piece of an HLA gene in their genome on chro-mosome 6. This small region, referred to as the* shared epitope, *contributes to the building of a protein that presents antigens to T cells. In other words, this gene piece seems to contribute to making those people more susceptible to RA.*

This gene segment is present in over half of all people with RA. Also, those individuals who inherit two copies of this gene segment have the most severe form of RA. One possible (as yet unproven) explanation for all this is that during inflammation in the joints, having the shared epitope may allow the presentation of self antigens like collagen or other cartilage molecules. That could excite the T cells to trigger an attack against the joint tissues, thinking that the self antigens were instead a sign of outside aggressors.

There is another hypothesis concerning the role of HLA genes in RA. There is evidence that they may influence that process in the thymus, the large gland in the upper chest where the young T cells are "educated" to not recognize the body's own tissues as dangerous, and trigger an immune response, as happens in RA. The hypothesis states that due to certain HLA genes some T cells that do recognize these self antigens escape from the thymus instead of being eliminated as they ordinarily would be.

Whatever the explanation, it is important to realize that while this shared epitope may be part of the genetic basis of RA in many people, it is by no means the whole story. For example, in African Americans, this gene segment is associ-ated with relatively few cases of RA. However, within any pop-ulation, people who do have the epitope, if they also have the "rheumatoid factor" in their blood, are thirteen times more likely to have severe RA.

Another genetic risk factor for RA is having a specific vari-ation of the gene that is in charge of making TNF-alpha, the cytokine chemical that is so active in the inflammation and damage in RA. A 1999 study showed that the most severe forms of RA in the people examined were found in those who had both that particular TNF-alpha gene and the shared epitope.

Of even more potential significance than the shared epitope may be the discovery of a form of gene that appears to be commonly associated with severe RA. In late 2000, scientists associated with the Vancouver General Hospital, Vancouver, British Columbia (www.vanhosp.bc.ca), announced that they had found a particular form of a gene that controls the production of the inflammatory cytokine *interferon-gamma* (*IFN-gamma*) by T cells in 73 percent of people with severe RA, compared to 21 percent with mild disease. This could lead the way to a deeper understanding of RA disease progression, help to predict the severity of an individual's RA, and help in guiding therapy.

Among genetic risk factors for RA, being female is certainly high on the list. Autoimmune diseases affect over 8.5 million people in the United States. Of these, 6.7 million are women. In RA (and multiple sclerosis) the female to male-ratio is between 2-to-1 and 3-to-1. The reasons for this gender gap are not clear. The U.S. National Multiple Sclerosis Society convened a task force of scientists to offer guidelines toward solving the question surrounding the gender basis of autoimmune diseases, including RA. The summary of their 1998 report is available at www.sciencemag.org/feature/data/983519.shl.

Female sex hormones appear to be associated with a greater risk for developing RA; the onset of the disease and painful flare-ups of symptoms are more frequent after childbirth, during lactation, and around menopause. In contrast, RA symptoms often lessen during pregnancy, and oral contraceptives have the same effect. The picture is by no means clear, however, in regard to gender. For example, RA that extends beyond the joints, such as rheumatoid lung disease, is far more common in men, while women require more hand and foot surgery due to RA.

There are several ways in which sex hormones could influence immune reactions. They could affect T cells or antigen-presenting cells, or help turn certain genes on or off. At this point there is no clear evidence concerning the precise basis for gender differences in autoimmunity. It is possible that gender differences could have implications for the timing and type of therapy—including the question of using sex hormones for treatment of autoimmune disease.

Testing for HLA genes typically is done when looking for compatible donors for tissue and organ transplants. Nonetheless, searching for specific HLA genes relative to RA has not been routine, because finding the genes does not necessarily mean that the person has the disease. However, it may become more common to test for RA-associated HLA genes, and now perhaps for the specific IFN-gamma gene type, in order to identify people who are at a greater risk for severe forms of RA at an early stage. This could lead to early aggressive treatment, which we now know can slow down the progression of RA. In 1999 a Japanese research group reported that they could routinely identify the RA-associated genes in question simply by taking fingernail clippings from people with RA and extracting and analyzing the DNA, avoiding the need for even taking blood samples.

The study of RA genetics has revealed more examples of the similarity and difference between RA and juvenile rheumatoid arthritis (JRA). JRA is also considered to be a complex, genetically influenced disease. While it also is often associated with the presence of HLA genes, unlike in RA, it is very rare for more than one member of a family to develop the disease. The incidence and prevalence of JRA also varies widely among different ethnic and geographically separate populations across the world. Early-onset pauciarticular

JRA—the type in which less than four joints are affected—makes up at least half of the diagnoses among Caucasians. It is rare among people of African and Asian descent. This suggests genetic differences in disease susceptibility. In terms of gender, the gap is even wider than in RA—this form of JRA occurs in a ratio of six to seven females for every male.

In 1994 the National Institute of Arthritis and Musculoskeletal and Skin Diseases (NIAMS; www.nih.gov/niams) awarded a contract to Children's Hospital Medical Center of Cincinnati, Ohio, to develop and maintain a research registry of people with JRA who have a biological sibling who also has JRA. The purpose of this registry is to locate people who might be willing to participate in research by investigators looking at the genetics of RA as well as other aspects of the disease.

It is clear that RA has a genetic component. While many individual researchers and their colleagues are now working to locate those genes, there are large-scale efforts underway as well. In response to the challenge of identifying RA-associated genes, in 1998 the European Consortium on Rheumatoid Arthritis Families published the results of their genome analysis of over four hundred families. Not only did they confirm a significant linkage of RA with HLA genes, but they uncovered as well a second major susceptibility region for RA that is on chromosome 3, as opposed to the HLA genes that are on chromosome 6.

While this genetic screening adds to the growing body of evidence about RA genetics, larger-scale studies are needed. In response to this need, the National Institutes of Health (NIH) and the Arthritis Foundation joined in establishing the North American Rheumatoid Arthritis Consortium (NARAC) in 1997. A group of twelve centers in the United States is collecting data from families containing sibling pairs affected by RA. By mid-2000 NARAC had enlisted eight hundred such families in this largest RA genetic study ever undertaken. The purpose is to identify specific sites on the chromosomes that appear to confer susceptibility to RA.

The researchers are examining DNA from the participants for approximately 350 different bits of genetic material that might identify any chromosomal regions that could harbor genes conferring susceptibility to RA. This project, while it will not identify specific RA genes, will narrow the search for these genes. It is as though they are looking for a few houses (the actual genes) somewhere in the United States, and are gradually narrowing the hunt down to the level of which states or even which cities within those states. The identification of the streets and finally the "houses" will then depend on the concerted efforts of many scientists who will be given access to the data generated in the NARAC project. NARAC offers detailed clinical information on the families—coded to preserve confidentiality. There are several levels of access to the site, and qualified investigators will have access to technical information and DNA samples.

The NARAC project is headed by Peter Gregersen, M.D., of North Shore University Hospital in Manhasset, New York. This endeavor, expected to be completed by 2003, will require the cooperation of rheumatologists and volunteers throughout the country. *A national toll-free number (1-800-382-4827) and e-mail address (narac@nshs.edu) are available to encourage participation.* The NARAC Web site lists the eligibility criteria for families who might wish to volunteer to take part in this study. The sites across the country that are members of the Consortium are found at www.medicine.ucsf.edu/narac.

    ✪   ✪   ✪

Are there perhaps genes that are common to many or all autoimmune diseases? So far, genetic analyses show that chromosome regions linked to autoimmunity are not randomly distributed across the genome but tend to cluster in at least eighteen regions. To look further at this important question, in September 1999 the National Institute of Allergy and Infectious Diseases (NIAID; www.niaid.nih.gov) announced plans to gather a large number of families in which several autoimmune diseases occur. This will include families with RA as well as, for example, lupus, type I diabetes, and multiple sclerosis. For more information on this project, the Multiple Autoimmune Disease Genetics Consortium (MADGC) has a Web site at www.madgc.org.

THE FINAL ANALYSIS

In October 1999 scientists hailed the announcement that the entire HLA complex, that stretch of DNA that makes the proteins that give our immune systems the capacity to distinguish "self" from "nonself," had been "sequenced" through the combined efforts of the Sanger Centre near Cambridge, England, the University of Washington in Seattle, and Tokai University in Japan. This means that by using powerful tools of DNA analysis, they determined the identity and the sequence of all 3,838,986 bases that make up that particular segment of chromosome 6. A visit to their Web site at www.sanger.ac.uk/HGP/Chr6/MHC.shtml leads to the sequence—simply a list of page after page of A, T, G, and C bases.

What might seem to be a boring list of almost 4 million letters is quite the opposite. It is a veritable treasure chest of information. The key to its usefulness has to do with the way proteins are made by cells. We have already pointed out that the sequence of bases in DNA determines the sequence of the amino acid building blocks in the proteins. More precisely, specific three-base sequences in the DNA determine the position of each of the twenty amino acids in a protein. In other words, when the cell makes a protein according to the commands of a gene, as the cell stitches amino acids together in a long, continuous chain, a base sequence of AGT might add amino acid #6, and the next sequence of CGA might add amino acid #12, and so on, until thousands of the amino acid building blocks become a protein with its own unique sequence and shape.

This genetic code is at the very heart of how all cells in the living world function according to directions from their genes. Genes are DNA, which is a sequence of bases. That base sequence determines the amino acid sequence in the protein that the gene orders the cell to make. The proteins go on to perform their assigned functions. And life goes on, driven by genes, which themselves are turned on and off by chemical signals.

One practical implication of the relationship between DNA bases and amino acid sequences in proteins is that if we know one, we can (with certain limitations) infer the other. That is, knowing the HLA base sequence can lead us to a better understanding of which proteins the HLA can make, and identifying a protein amino acid sequence (easily done in a modern laboratory) can tell us what kind of DNA was in charge of making that protein. In terms of RA, for example, knowing the exact base sequence of the genes in the HLA can help lead us to the proteins that it makes—and eventually, we hope, to some control over those genes and proteins. The same, of course, can be said of the search for the genes that are in charge of making the cytokines, those chemical messengers that drive the immune system.

The exciting possibilities for locating genes and their protein products and for devising healing and preventive therapies based on that knowledge will be realized as individual gene research efforts meld with the Human Genome Project. This latter massive project began in 1990, cosponsored by the

Department of Energy and the National Institutes of Health as a $3-billion, proposed fifteen-year effort to determine the DNA base sequence of the human genome and, in so doing, to eventually lead to the identification of all the estimated thirty to forty thousand human genes. By 2000 it had become an eighteen-nation international effort from the United States to Europe to Japan and China.

The sequence information, updated on a daily basis, and related nontechnical Human Genome Project information is available at www.sanger.ac.uk/HGP or ornl.gov/hgmis. Scientists from academia and industry are free to scan and use the information. Tens of thousands of genes have already been identified from the genome sequence, including genes responsible for dozens of inherited diseases such as epilepsy, diabetes, hereditary deafness, cystic fibrosis, and Duchenne muscular dystrophy.

The atlas of the base sequences in the human genome has begun to revolutionize biological research and medical practice at this early stage of the twenty-first century. Eventually, all human genes will be found, leading to early, accurate diagnosis and therapy of many diseases. Now that most of the genome sequence is known, the challenge has just begun. The crucial question is, exactly where along that sequence of billions of bases stretched along the DNA strands are each of the genes—and what do each of them do?

In what is literally a competitive race to find those genes, the Human Genome Project is by no means the only player in what has been dubbed the "genome gold rush." It is possible to secure patents on the use of genes for commercial purposes, and in developing diagnostics and treatments the possibilities for profit are enormous. One leader in this effort is Celera Genomics in Rockville, Maryland, headed by Craig Venter, formerly at NIH. Celera (www.celera.com), using a sequencing technique different from that utilized in the Human Genome

Project, and integrating the free published results with their own data, claimed to have sequenced almost the entire genome by mid-2000. Dr. Venter says that his company will make money by "helping our clients interpret that data."

What literally became an acrimonious race between Celera and the Human Genome Project to complete the genome sequencing ended in a somewhat uneasy truce in mid-2000. At a White House press conference on June 26, cohosted by President Clinton and Prime Minister Tony Blair, the two sides made a joint announcement that they had effectively sequenced almost the entire genome. Then, in February 2001, Celera and the Human Genome Project simultaneously published their massive genome sequencing results.

In addition, Celera had completed sequencing the entire mouse genome by early 2001. Mice and humans are separated by 100 million years of evolution, but our genomes are about the same size, and most human genes have counterparts in the mouse genome. (The query, "Are you a man or a mouse?" is no longer a scientifically valid question.) Knowledge of the mouse genome sequence will help identify the role of human genes. Scientists studying a human gene can locate the mouse counterpart, create a strain of mouse that lacks that gene, and find out what the effects are on the mouse. Celera's mouse genome will be available to paid subscribers.

Another example of the hunt for treasure in the human genome is the exploration underway in Newfoundland and Labrador. The province's population of approximately 555,000 —descended from a small number of immigrant ancestors, making it easier to check families for shared genes—has an increased prevalence of such autoimmune diseases as psoriasis, diabetes, and RA. Newfoundland Genetics, a partnership between the British biotechnology company, Gemini Holdings plc, Cambridge, U.K. (www.gemini-genomics.com), and Lineage Biomedical Inc., St. John's, Newfoundland, began to search this population in 2000 to identify genes that might predispose people to these diseases, with the hope of patenting and profiting from the commercial use of those genes as well as helping those who have the diseases. They have agreed to direct some revenues to an independent, not-for-profit foundation for Newfoundlanders with diseases traced to the gene discoveries.

Other companies, concentrating on the proteins rather than the genes, have created a new field called proteomics. Their aim is to isolate and analyze all possible human proteins—with emphasis on those that might be useful in disease treatment. International Business Machines Corp. (IBM), Armonk, New York (www.ibm.com), is building a supercomputer five hundred times more powerful than any current computer, which they will use to analyze proteins to help design effective medications, perhaps even custom designed to the needs of individual people.

There are many controversies over the accuracy of the gene sequences from sources other than the Human Genome Project, the ethics of patenting human genes, the commercialization of the human genome, and other related issues. The fact remains that gene-based medicine will only expand rapidly as more and more genes are pinpointed, their precise functions in the body are discovered, and therapies are designed to give us greater control over disease and suffering.

We are gaining a clearer focus on the emerging, still hazy picture of the contributions of genes to RA. What type of gene-centered therapies are researchers already considering and testing in the fight against RA? Let's look at some exciting new developments that offer hope.

CHAPTER 5

By Means of Genes

O ur genes, all thirty to forty thousand or so of them (although that number is still a rough estimate), lie scattered at intervals along the length of the tightly coiled chromosomes deep inside each of our body's cells, nestled within a membrane-bound sac: the nucleus. There, far away from the watery mix of chemicals bathing the outer surface of the cells that harbor the chromosomes, some of the genes periodically switch on—directing the cell to make specific proteins—and then switch off. Each cell has a complete complement of genes—the full set of instructions to make a complete human—and yet at any one time only a fraction of the genes are active, ordering the cells to fashion only the proteins needed at that particular time and place.

We know that among all those genes there are some that make us susceptible to developing RA. We have pinpointed some of those genes and will doubtless soon track down others. We also know that the continuing painful inflammation and joint damage so characteristic of RA is brought about by means of chemical messenger proteins, the cytokines, such as IL-1 and TNF-alpha, as well as other destructive proteins, the enzymes that gradually erode cartilage and bone.

The Human Genome Project and many other large and

more modest research efforts are coalescing in painting a clearer picture of where these genes are located on the chromosomes and even the exact sequence of their molecular building blocks. But even when we know precisely where genes are and what their exact sequence is, how can we possibly get at those tiny bits of DNA? After all, they are buried in a tangled mass of thousands of other different genes, packed away in each of the trillions of cells that make up the human body. And if we can somehow contact them, how can we affect what they do? Can we do something to turn them on or off, speed up their activity or slow them down, or, to be even more far-fetched, could we even dream of being able to "repair" genes that we might discover are defective? Might this be a way to control or stop the destruction wrought by RA, by reaching into the deepest recesses of the cells and influencing the genes behind the disease?

As a matter of fact, since the 1970s, a gradual development of innovative methods for locating, extracting, and manipulating genes has led to sophisticated techniques that have answered a qualified "yes" to each of the above questions. We are now at the beginning of a new era of medicine based on using genes themselves as prime therapeutic targets.

According to W. French Anderson, the brilliant physician whose pioneering research contributed so much to the birth of this new age of *genetic engineering*, there have been four major revolutions in medicine since Hippocrates first argued, some twenty-four hundred years ago, that the functions of the body can be explained by laws of nature, difficult though it might be to determine those laws. The first revolution occurred after British surgeon John Snow discovered, in 1854, that cholera, a devastating and frequently fatal intestinal infection, is spread by water contaminated with human waste. This led to the use of sanitation systems that have saved people from cholera and other devastating infections that have plagued humankind.

The second revolution, which evolved at about the same time, was surgery with anesthesia, and the third revolution was the introduction of vaccines (beginning in the late nineteenth century) and antibiotics, starting with penicillin in the early 1940s. The fourth medical revolution, according to Anderson and echoed by many scientists, will be the development and use of of human genetic engineering, otherwise known as *gene therapy*, first applied to a human with partial success by Anderson and his colleagues in 1990.

In terms of gene-based treatments for disease, as the twenty-first century begins, we are only in the very early stages of what promises to be a sweeping revolution in medicine. In the space of a few years, gene therapy has passed from being a distant ideal in the minds of a few pioneers to a subject of intense experimentation. Within a few decades many think that most diseases will probably have some form of gene manipulation as a treatment option. This will include inserting genes into people to substitute for genes that are absent or not working properly and treating genes with drugs that will target and modify their function. Biotechnology and pharmaceutical companies are making major commitments to research and development in both of these approaches.

Genetic modifications are not limited to genes that are driving human diseases. All organisms, from bacteria to humans, are gene-based living systems. There are frequent reports in the media announcing the latest genetically altered animals and plants, now referred to as genetically-modified organisms (GMOs). These alterations range from the genetic engineering of goats so that they produce pharmaceuticals in their milk, to the addition of genes to pigs so that their organs might someday be compatible for transplanting into humans, to the genetic modification of foods such as corn or wheat that are given new genes in order to render them resistant to herbicides or disease.

Controversies surround almost every aspect of genetic manipulation. There are concerns over the safety of consuming genetically altered plants, and ethical questions about subjecting humans and animals to certain kinds of genetic experimentation. All of these are significant and valid subjects for careful discussion. However, our interest here is in the window of opportunity opened up by this new era that may lead to fascinating possibilities for prevention, treatment, or perhaps even cure of RA.

The Gene Machine

Genes do not act on their own. We are discovering, piece by piece, a dynamic system that monitors, controls, and fine-tunes their operations. Our growing understanding of this system does more than just satisfy our intellectual curiosity. An automobile mechanic needs to understand the workings of spark plugs, pistons, fuel injectors, and a car's electrical circuits, and how all of those parts and many others interact to make the engine run smoothly. Anyone who wants to "tune up" living cells so that they hum along in perfect health needs to know how all the parts of those cells relate to each other in health and in disease. Of course, when an automobile breaks down, sometimes trial and error can get it back on the road. Maybe the unlucky driver who otherwise knows little about engines can tighten a loose fan belt or add water to a thirsty radiator and get moving again.

We may not like to admit it, but some medical treatments, even though they are sometimes effective, are based on the same serendipitous approach as that of the stranded driver. The treatments are not always based on a precise knowledge of how a drug actually influences the inner workings of our cells. That certainly is true of some medications used for RA (see chapter 7). As long as they are safe and give some relief, we are grateful to use them. However, a better understanding of their effects can warn us against possible dangers in their long-term use, help us to modify them to sharpen their effectiveness, and give us clues for creating better and safer medications. Also, what works for one individual may not help another.

We have made amazing progress in our understanding of how genes work and how to work with genes, even though we still have a long way to go. We can extract DNA from cells and isolate specific genes from that mass of DNA. Once the genes are isolated, they can be copied millions of times by putting them into microorganisms like bacteria or yeast, which will faithfully replicate them each time the cells divide. Or, they can be incubated with a supply of DNA building blocks and enzymes in a laboratory device (the PCR machine) where they will copy themselves over and over.

Genes, once remote, inaccessible bits of DNA, can now be identified, isolated from cells, and copied into whatever quantities are needed. Minute amounts of those genes can be put into the cells of living organisms where, amazingly, the genes will often enter the nucleus, latch onto and become part of the chromosomes, and function as though they were meant to be there. This process of adding functional genes to cells, called *genetic transformation*, is the reason why we are now able to make so many different genetically modified organisms. Almost all GMOs are now at the research stage and not cleared for commercial use. However a few, like corn, wheat, and soybeans, are now widely used in agriculture, and many other modified plants and animals are waiting in the wings.

How is it possible to put genes, minute DNA molecules, into cells so small that they are invisible to the naked eye? There are a number of ways to do just that, but we will concentrate on the methods devised over the last twenty years to get functional genes into animal (including human) cells. The ultimate goal is to bring about a gene-based therapeutic result—the transfer of genes to people so that the genes will express proteins that will treat or cure illnesses.

To do that, we need some kind of *vector*, something that can carry the genes into the target cells. Sometimes genes can be introduced into cells by wrapping them in tiny spheres of fatty material called *liposomes*. These will soak through cell membranes, carrying their DNA cargo inside. There, as we have pointed out, in a small percentage of cases the genes will incorporate themselves into the cell's chromosomes and become part of the cell's genome. DNA can even be coated onto microscopic gold particles and literally shot into cells using a device known as a gene gun.

In most of the instances that pertain to human RA research, DNA carriers have been kindly provided by nature in the form of viruses. Viruses are not living organisms. So small that they cannot be seen even with the ordinary laboratory microscope, they are merely bits of RNA or DNA wrapped in a bit of protein. They can propagate themselves only by entering a living cell and taking it over, forcing it to make viral copies. To use viruses as vectors, researchers disable the parts of the viral genetic instructions that allow the viruses to replicate in living cells, and wrap the genes that they want to transfer inside the virus protein coat. Then, when the viruses are mingled with cells—perhaps in a test tube in the laboratory, or inside an animal or human joint —the viruses will slip into those cells, releasing the experimental genes.

Gene therapy experiments use a variety of viral types, each of which has advantages and disadvantages. One of the real challenges in developing an efficient means of gene therapy for RA, or any other disease, is in devising a vector—viral or otherwise—that is safe and effective.

What about human gene therapy? During the 1990s there were almost four hundred *clinical trials* using genetic manipulations related to treating human diseases carried out with more than four thousand human volunteers (see chapter 9 for an explanation of clinical trials). Most of the procedures were of the gene-addition variety. The researchers attempted to put normal genes into cells that harbored defective forms of those genes. By 2000 there were six thousand people in three dozen countries undergoing gene therapy experiments. Most of the procedures were aimed at cancer, but included at least twenty-two other conditions, including cystic fibrosis, hemophilia, coronary artery disease, AIDS—and three trials of gene therapy for RA.

Savio L. C. Woo, Ph.D., president of the American Society of Gene Therapy (www.asgt.org), reflected the state of the art of human gene therapy in general when he addressed twenty-five hundred delegates at the 2000 annual meeting. "Gene therapy," said Dr. Woo, "is in its infancy as a biomedical discipline. We are already seeing preliminary results, through clinical trials, that give us glimpses of hope that we will be able to offer effective treatments for debilitating and often deadly diseases . . . it's finally coming together."

In fact, a few months earlier, in April of 2000, Dr. Alain Fischer and his colleagues at Necker Children's Hospital in Paris (www.anapath.necker.fr) published the results of the first unequivocal success of human gene therapy. Three babies who lacked the genes to make a complete immune system were given genes that transformed their immune systems into normal, working systems, capable of fending off infections that might otherwise prove fatal to them. Their very rare disease, a form of "severe combined immune deficiency," or SCID, presents an ideal target for gene therapy. These babies are born with a nonfunctioning gene normally used to make T cells, those white blood cells central to the normal functioning of the immune system (and which, as we have seen, appear to be the driving force behind the destruction in RA).

The researchers removed bone marrow from each baby, treated the marrow so that some of the bone marrow cells accepted a dose of normal T cell genes, and placed the marrow back into the baby. There the genetically corrected cells proliferated, replacing those cells in the marrow with the defective genes, and triggered the production of millions of healthy T cells.

In spite of the enthusiasm created by this remarkable achievement, the current status of human gene therapy is that it is still too inefficient to be helpful for most diseases. After the SCID research, the most promising trials have been in stimulating new blood vessel growth in the heart to treat heart failure or in the limbs to repair limited circulation. Other promising discoveries reported at the American Society of Gene Therapy meeting offered innovative approaches to hemophilia and some forms of cancer.

✛   ✛   ✛

So far, most gene therapy techniques aimed at human diseases have been of the gene-addition variety. These are attempts to get normal genes into cells that have malfunctioning genes. Challenging though this may be, it is in a sense a straightforward problem. Diseases like cystic fibrosis, hemophilia, sickle-cell disease, and muscular dystrophy are of the "single-gene" variety. Each can be traced to a specific gene that has been identified and for which the normal form of the gene can be prepared in the laboratory. Even under these conditions, there are still major obstacles to overcome in finding just the right methods for getting the corrective genes into ailing cells, and seeing to it that the therapeutic genes behave reliably and at beneficial levels.

The challenge is even more formidable for therapeutic gene modifications of diseases where the genetic picture is not so clear—as in the case of diabetes, Alzheimer's, cancer, or RA. To understand the therapeutic opportunities arising from the work of the many researchers now trying to meet those challenges, particularly with regard to RA, we need to get back to the basics of how genes go about their business, in order to intervene for our own healing purposes.

GENE BASICS

Genes are in charge of making proteins. They do not actually stitch together the long chains of amino acids that form the proteins. That assembly is done outside the nucleus, on the surface of roughly spherical granules, the ribosomes, which are scattered throughout the cell. Each cell has thousands of these granules, scenes of a constant buzz of activity as proteins are put together and sent off to various parts of the cell to fulfill their appointed tasks. The sequence of the thousands of building blocks making up the genes, called *bases*, signified by the initials A, T, G, or C, determines the sequence of thousands of the twenty different amino acid building blocks in the proteins.

How is the knowledge of the gene base sequence transmitted to the ribosomes? A copy of the gene (actually a mirror image) is made, in the form of another molecule called RNA. This "messenger" RNA, carrying the information about the base sequence of the gene, moves out to the ribosomes, drapes across them, and the protein chains are assembled one amino acid at a time along the length of the messenger RNA, according to its particular base sequence.

The process of making the RNA, the faithful messenger carrying the genetic code for protein manufacture, is known as *transcription*. Here is where controls operate that make it possible for the cell to be a fine-tuned, organized, dynamic living entity. In any given cell, there are lots of genes that are always turned on, sending off messenger RNA to make proteins that the cell needs to have in constant supply. However, for most genes, there is a strict set of controls that regulate their activity.

Most genes do not get transcribed, that is, they cannot make a length of messenger RNA and send it off to make proteins, unless the genes receive specific signals to do so. Those signals vary widely and can be environmental (e.g., temperature or light) or internal (e.g., hormones or cytokines). As we saw in chapter 2, a cell knows what is going on outside of it only when it receives and interprets chemical cues that arrive at its outer border, the delicate cell membrane. One category of such cues includes chemicals that turn genes on or off.

How is it possible to switch genes on and off? First, let's look a little more closely at the gene. It turns out that a gene includes not only a stretch of DNA that can be transcribed into messenger RNA, but another piece of DNA next to that called the *promoter*, almost like a trigger needed to "fire" the gene. When a chemical signal arrives at the cell membrane, it attaches to a compatible protein receptor on the membrane, like a hand fitting into a glove. This sets off a cascade of chemical reactions inside the cell—the products of one reaction trigger the next reaction and so on—resulting in the production of specific chemicals called *transcription factors*. A transcription factor binds to a particular site promoter, and turns on the gene (Fig. 11). It's the concept of the assembly line again—one step leads to the next, which leads to the next, and then finally the finished product—an active gene. *This step-by-step process, starting with the cell receiving a signal and ending with a turned-on gene, is a key target for experimental genetic regulation of RA.*

We know that the prolonged progression of RA, once established, appears to take on a momentum of its own. Inflammation may be slowed down by medications, but not stopped. Now that we are learning more about the transcription factors that play a central role in activating the genes behind the scenes, we are searching for ways to gain control over them.

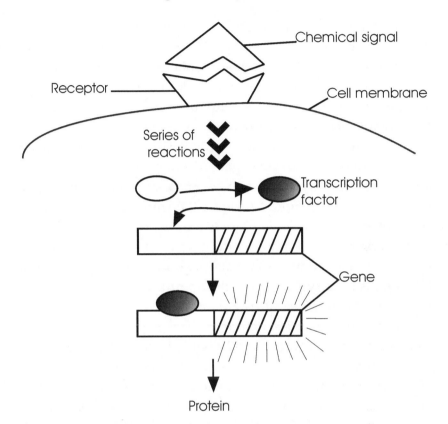

Fig. 11. Genes can be "turned on" to make a protein. A chemical signal is received by a protein receptor on the cell surface. This sets off a series of chemical reactions in the cell, resulting in a transcription factor literally becoming attached to the DNA. This in turn activates a particular gene to give directions to the cell to make a specific protein (see Fig. 9).

Almost inadvertently, physicians have been doing that to a certain extent already. We now know that several of the medications (chapter 7) long used to treat RA act in part by blocking the activity of certain transcription factors. The medications sulfasalazine, gold compounds, and glucocorticoids (steroids) all inhibit one of the transcription factors central to inflammation. There are at least four groups of transcription factors that operate in RA. The specific factor influenced by the above, nuclear factor kappaB (NF-kappaB) deserves particular emphasis because it is a pivotal regulator of inflammation.

NF-kappaB turns on the genes that make TNF-alpha and IL-1, those cytokines that perpetuate inflammation. In RA both of these cytokines are major driving forces behind the abnormal enlargement of the synovial membrane lining the joints, leading to erosion of cartilage and bone. Another one of the effects that those cytokines have is to stimulate cells in the joint to make even more NF-kappaB, forming a vicious cycle of inflammation. The effects of this transcription factor reach even further. It even has a hand in helping to make molecules that assist in attracting and grabbing onto inflammatory white blood cells as they pass through the minute blood vessels surrounding the joint, recruiting them to join the attack.

There are therapies now in the testing and development stage that strike directly at TNF-alpha and IL-1 (chapter 10). But given that these destructive cytokines are manufactured by genes that are literally turned on by the transcription factor NF-kappaB, it would seem logical to try to block that factor before the genes could be activated by it. If you are bothered by the light, why not dismantle the light switch?

This is an approach that shows some promise for RA therapy. Researchers at the Kennedy Institute of Rheumatology in London (www.arc.org.uk/common/home.htm), fighting fire with fire so to speak, have managed to turn on genes that make a potent suppressor of NF-kappaB. Halfway around the world, at the Osaka University Medical School in Japan (www.med.osaka-u.ac.jp), scientists have blocked NF-kappaB by using pieces of DNA designed to latch onto the NF-kappaB, inactivating it before it gets a chance to turn on genes. These approaches to blocking harmful gene products such as cytokines at the very source of their manufacture may become a very useful tool in the management of RA.

These new strategies for blocking transcription factors (and the above are only a few examples out of many experiments) are not the only points along the assembly line of inflammation that are under scrutiny. Specific gene discoveries offer even more therapeutic possibilities. For example, researchers at the Weizmann Institute of Science in Rehovot, Israel (www.weizmann.ac.il), announced in 1999 that they had isolated a gene responsible for making a protein that might help block autoimmune diseases. The protein, called IL-18BP, blocks the operations of yet another cytokine with multiple inflammatory effects, IL-18. Because they could reproduce the gene in the laboratory they were able to make enough IL-18BP to show this effect when it was injected into mice.

In that same year, researchers at Boston University School of Dental Medicine in Boston, Massachusetts (dentalschool.bu.edu), reported the identification of a gene that plays a role in controlling production of TNF-alpha. This gene, known as LITAF, helps to turn on another gene that makes TNF-alpha. This gene is a new member of the growing list of therapeutic targets aimed at lowering the levels of this central cytokine.

Soon after the LITAF discovery, a team at the biotechnology firm Celltech Chiroscience in Seattle (www.chiroscience.com) announced their discovery of a gene in both mice and humans, which they called the scurfy gene. It regulates some of the harmful activities of T cells, that cell type central to many immune responses.

So the list of gene-based possibilities for RA therapy grows. It is important to emphasize that these discoveries that we have summarized so far have all been made using either living animals or animal or human cells that were growing in laboratory cultures. The experiments are conducted on animals (not humans) whose specific human disease symptoms are induced by a wide variety of stimuli. These include selective breeding, subjecting them to various chemicals, or manipulating their genes in some way. In the latter case we now have ingenious techniques for inserting a gene of choice into the chromosomes of an animal. A batch of the genes are injected into a fertilized egg, and the egg develops with some of the added genes now an integral part of the animals genome. The animal, now referred to as *transgenic*, expresses that gene along with its normal genes.

This kind of gene insertion is random, however, and the new gene may in fact sometimes end up disrupting a normal gene. To avoid that potential problem, and to zero in on specific genes in the animal's genome, one can now apply gene targeting. This technique actually inserts the gene into a specific site on the chromosome, replacing a targeted gene. This approach has created a whole new generation of experimental subjects referred to as *knockout animals*, because a gene has literally been "knocked out" of their genome.

Many different species of animals, large and small, serve as valuable subjects in the search to uncover the details of what goes on in the cells, tissues, and organs during human diseases as well as for testing the effects of treatments aimed at those disorders. That is certainly true in RA research, including gene-based research.

We will forgo any discussion here about the controversies that invariably surround the use of animals in research. There are those who object strenuously to subjecting animals to the pain and discomfort that often accompany medical experimentation. If one were to ask average citizens whether or not we should ban the utilization of animals for tests that stood a good chance of enabling us to find a more effective treatment or cure for rheumatoid arthritis, or perhaps a vaccine against AIDS, it seems reasonable to assume that most would support such experiments. Many would also emphasize that care should be taken to prevent needless suffering of the animals. In fact, there are strict federal regulations that require that animals must be treated in a humane way.

The preferred animals for studying RA are mice, rats, and rabbits. Mice and rats are the traditional experimental animals in the life sciences because they reproduce rapidly and are easy to handle; moreover, there is a lot of basic information available on their metabolism and genetics to serve as a frame of reference. A female mouse, for example, can produce a dozen babies only three months after her own birth. The greater size of rabbits make them particularly useful in RA experiments where substances are injected into the joints.

The most important model for RA is the collagen-induced arthritis (CIA) mouse. The cartilage protein type II collagen, when injected into mice, causes them to develop an RA-like condition. Neither this model nor any other reflects all of the features of human RA. After all, these animals are separated from us by millions of years of evolutionary history—but intense examination of their genomes has revealed that their genetic makeup and tendency to arthritis bear many striking similarities to our own. Each model has contributed something to our understanding of the complicated mechanisms behind RA.

One very interesting result of creating RA animal models is that very different stimuli—chemical, bacterial, and genetic manipulations—can lead to RA symptoms in those animals. This underscores the fact that RA has come to be widely regarded as a syndrome, that is, a set of damaging symptoms in response to any number of different provoking factors.

Sometimes nature provides animal models by sheer serendipity. A well-known example is that of the SCID mice. These mice were discovered in 1980 in a litter that happened to be undergoing routine tests on the mouse immune system. The mice had inherited a pair of mutant genes, which meant that they could not make a key enzyme necessary to build up a functional immune system. Because of that, they lacked T and B cells, for example. The mice were interbred and their thousands of descendants have been used in research not only on the human form of SCID, but for studies on transplantation and many diseases like AIDS and RA.

One reason that these SCID mice are so useful is that, since they lack a normal immune system, one can put cells into them from other organisms, including humans, and the recipients will not have the immune system tools to reject them. For instance, in one series of experiments, cells from human synovium were removed from the joints of people with RA. The gene for making the cytokine IL-10 was put into the cells and they were then implanted into SCID mice along with pieces of human cartilage. Ordinarily the synovial cells would have invaded and destroyed the cartilage, but not in this case.

In other words, IL-10, known to be a cytokine chemical messenger that can inhibit the inflammatory effects of cytokines such as TNF-alpha and IL-1, was literally produced in such quantities in the genetically modified synovial cells that it had powerful anti-inflammatory effects. It might be feasible to put IL-10 genes into synovial cells in human joints to do the same thing. These kinds of experiments with the SCID mice have made it a highly useful animal model for evaluating treatment strategies.

Another approach utilizing synovial cells that may prove helpful has been used in rabbits. In that case, the genes were injected directly into the joints, where they took up residence in the synovial cells. The long-term goal is to alter synovial gene activity, inhibiting the role of the synovial cells, which ordinarily help to develop and maintain the progressive destruction of cartilage and bone in RA.

Other examples from what is becoming a long list of successful experiments are the creation of transgenic mice that are "humanized" in that they can make human antigens associated with RA, or the reduction of cartilage damage in mice joints after the mice were given genes for making the cytokine IL-4.

Also, destructive synovial cell growth in RA has been blocked in rats by injecting genes that make a growth-inhibiting enzyme.

In some animal gene therapy experiments, cells are taken from the animal and genes are put into the cells. Then the genetically transformed cells are put back into the subject. In other instances the experimenters inject the genes, usually in a vector, directly into the animal's joints. In either case the principle is the same—rather than give the animal the gene protein products directly, with limited success, why not insert the genes for making those proteins where they might succeed in taking up residence and supply the protein when and where it is needed?

An unexpected but welcome phenomenon has been observed during the course of several of these animal experiments. Injection of genes packaged in a virus vector into one knee joint of rabbit and mice RA models not only slows down the disease in the infected joint, but also in the opposite, untreated joint! This offers the hope that it might someday be possible to inject one arthritic joint in a person with RA and have other arthritic joints in the body respond—which brings us finally to the subject of RA gene therapy trials in humans.

HUMAN TRIALS

It's a long trek from the lab bench to the clinic. First, an idea is born in the mind of a scientist, perhaps merely a glimmer of hope for a new and useful approach to treat a human disease. The idea is based on an intimate knowledge of many other experiments that relate somehow to it—experiments published in any one of thousands of science journals—perhaps read in a library or online. The idea may have been sparked while hearing a report at a conference, or in a conversation with another researcher, or perhaps it came from an observation made in the scientist's own laboratory.

Whatever the source, the idea must be tested. Perhaps the initial experiments are done in test tubes or flasks of living cells, human or otherwise. If all goes well, the next step is to use animals. There are serious considerations to keep in mind, including the safety of the procedure, the required dosage, the best means of delivery, and a careful monitoring for side effects. If the research is carried out in a biotechnology company, funds, personnel, and equipment may be available for the investigation. If it occurs at a university and/or a medical center, considerable time and effort will go into applying for funding from private or, more often, federal government sources such as the National Institutes of Health (NIH).

Then, often years after the original concept was born, if the procedure has stood the test of time and the rigors of scientific scrutiny, the proposed therapy moves at last to the clinic, where human volunteers will agree to undergo testing. In the United States, human gene therapy, often referred to as human gene transfer research, is overseen jointly by the Food and Drug Administration (FDA) and the NIH. Within the research community, in each of the more than four thousand universities, hospitals, and other research institutions receiving federal funding there are special oversight committees, known as institutional review boards (IRBs), which are responsible for seeing to it that the investigators under their supervision adhere to all government standards. All human subjects, for one thing, must give their informed consent, meaning that they agree to the procedure only after being given all relevant information. This includes the nature of the procedure, the risks, the benefits, and the alternatives.

While the FDA actually approves gene transfer clinical trials, the NIH Recombinant DNA Advisory Committee (RAC) provides additional oversight and public discussion of those trials—including whatever ethical issues may arise, with the safety of the human subjects being the paramount issue. Since the formation of the Human Gene Therapy Subcommittee in 1984, all of the more than four hundred approved human gene transfer protocols had been aimed at diseases normally considered lethal—such as cancer, AIDS, and cystic fibrosis. On July 17, 1996, doctors at the University of Pittsburgh Medical Center (www.upmc.edu) began a clinical trial of gene therapy for RA, the first FDA-approved gene therapy trial for a nonlethal disease.

This, and the others described below, are all phase I clinical trials. That means that they are designed as the first, cautious steps leading toward possible application of the techniques for actual treatment of people suffering from a disease. Phase I trials are designed to test the safety of the procedure. Later trials, if phase I is deemed safe, are designed more toward proving that the procedures are actually therapeutic, and help determine the correct dosages.

Sixty-eight-year-old Carlene Lauffer had suffered from rheumatoid arthritis for twenty years. Her condition had advanced to the point where she faced surgery to replace her knuckles with artificial joints. In April of 1996, in a procedure developed by researchers Chris Evans and Paul Robbins and performed by orthopedic surgeon James Herndon, cells removed from the synovial membrane of one of her thumb joints were transferred to a sterile growth medium in the lab. The cells reproduced and some were modified to carry a gene that blocks inflammation.

On July 17, Herndon injected two of Lauffer's knuckle joints with gene-enhanced cells and two with untreated cells, to determine the difference. One week later, the surgeon removed Lauffer's knuckles and replaced them with artificial ones. They kept tissue and fluid from the joints to examine them to see if the genes had any beneficial effects. After this first groundbreaking experiment, eight other women over the next several years were treated in a similar manner.

All procedures had similar, welcome results. First, there

were no adverse effects seen. In addition, the researchers found that the injected cells containing the genes had not only survived but the genes functioned normally, and produced their protein product within the joint—giving support for the hope that genes delivered to arthritic joints might let the joints make their own medicine where it is needed most.

To be more specific about this modest but highly significant milestone in RA therapy history, the gene that they used, packaged in a harmless virus to get it into the synovial cells, was one that directs the synthesis of a naturally occurring immune system protein, interleukin-1 receptor antagonist (IL-1ra). This protein, produced in reponse to infection or inflammation, blocks the actions of what should now be a familiar cytokine, interleukin-1 (IL-1). This cytokine is made in large quantities in RA, in which case the IL-1ra, normally present in the tissues, does not seem to be able to do its usual job to sufficiently counter the IL-1 inflammatory effects. In fact, there is some evidence in animal experiments that some people with RA may not be able to make enough IL-1ra.

The IL-1 cytokine drives inflammation by first attaching to special receptor sites on the surface of joint cells. The IL-1ra can also attach to the same sites, like an automobile pulling into someone else's parking spot. When that happens, it blocks the cytokine from latching onto that site and starting trouble. While repeated injections of IL-1ra into animals and humans have shown some modest anti-inflammatory effects, the ideal situation would be to have the IL-1ra made by genes inside the joints threatened by RA.

These University of Pittsburgh experiments were not designed to treat RA in those particular nine individuals, but to ensure that the procedure is safe and to confirm that gene transfer to human joints is possible. Their protocol was the result of more than eight years of rigorous preparation. Now, having proven both safety and some degree of effectiveness, the next step will be to extend these approaches with other volunteers with less advanced disease in order to work toward the ideal of gene therapy for RA.

During the time of the Pittsburgh clinical trials, researchers at the University of Dusseldorf in Germany (www.rz.uni-duesseldorf.de), in collaboration with the Pittsburgh group, began using a similar experimental approach. Their approach differed in that the gene-bearing cells were inserted into the joints one month, rather than one week, before surgery. By mid-2000 they had used their procedure with two people, and had results similar to those in the larger Pittsburgh trial—there were no adverse effects, and the genes in the injected cells functioned properly.

In the third and only other RA gene therapy experiments done to date with humans, a team led by Blake Roessler at the University of Michigan Medical Center (www.med.umich.edu/1welcome/index1.htm) began, in August 1999, a phase I clinical trial in which they tested a technique often used with promising results in cancer gene therapy trials. This procedure uses a gene taken from a virus. The gene, when injected into living tissues, enters some of the cells and causes them to make an enzyme, TK, which normally is not present in human cells. Then gancyclovir, a drug harmless to normal human cells, is given to the person. In cells that have produced TK, the gancyclovir is converted to a toxic substance that kills only those TK-producing cells.

The ultimate aim of using this approach for RA would be as a means of shrinking the pannus—that inflamed, enlarged, encroaching, destructive growth of the normally delicate and protective synovial membrane lining the joints. Perhaps this growth can be slowed by getting many of its cells to die under the influence of the TK-gancyclovir interaction, as though they had been poisoned. By mid-2000 two volunteers had undergone injections of the TK gene into their knee joints safely and with evidence that cells that expressed the TK gene in their inflamed synovial membranes had been destroyed by the gancyclovir treatment. The researchers plan on repeating the experiment with six additional volunteers.

✚   ✚   ✚

In looking at the positive and promising results coming out of these early steps along the road to gene therapy for RA, it's important to keep in mind that it may very well be that blocking the effects of a single inflammatory cytokine such as IL-1, for example, may not be sufficient. Synovial cells could still play a central role in cartilage damage under the influence of other genes such as those that make cartilage dissolving enzymes or those that make molecules that help the aggressive synovial cells stick to cartilage. That is why a means of inactivating the synovial cells, such as by means of TK genes, could be of critical importance by eliminating many of those cells that are so influential in RA.

In other words, it looks as though stopping joint destruction in RA, whether it is by the means described above or others that are sure to come along, will require interference with more than one step in the assembly line that is putting together a multifaceted attack on those joints. Gene therapy may prove to be a powerful ally in that blockade.

Promising though it is, the use of genes as tools and targets in the fight against RA is in its infancy. Nevertheless, the potential seems great, and the possibilities are wide-reaching. That is true as well for our next topic. Scientists are beginning to use primitive, unspecialized cells found throughout the body—the *stem cells*—as a means of rebuilding tissues damaged by disease—including the immune system.

CHAPTER 6

Stemming the Tide

The bones of our skeletal system are by no means simply dead and rigid attachment sites for our muscles, tendons, and ligaments. Nor are they "just" a protective framework for internal organs. They are, in fact, dynamic living tissues that can grow, adapt to stress, and repair themselves after injury. Every bone is a rich, dense matrix of collagen protein and minerals, mainly calcium phosphate, that envelops millions of living bone cells. These cells lie buried within minute cavities in the bone. The cavities are connected to each other by a complex series of microscopic canals, used for carrying nutrition and waste disposal. Bone has an abundant blood supply, important not only for nourishing the buried cells, but also for communicating with the bone's hollow interior.

There, protected by heavy surrounding walls, is the *bone marrow*: a rich, pulpy mass of tissue vital to our survival. Yellow marrow, which is mostly fatty tissue, fills the large cavity in the shafts of the long bones, like the femur of the leg, or the humerus in the upper arm. More important is the red marrow, packed into the honeycombed ends of the long bones, and filling the interior of many other bones such as the pelvis and the sternum, the flat breastbone in the center of the chest.

Here in the red marrow special cells divide by the millions each second of our lives, replenishing our blood cells. Blood is actually a type of *connective tissue*, consisting of cells within a liquid, the blood plasma, which circulates through the heart and blood vessels. The blood carries vital nutrients to our other tissues and removes the waste products of their metabolism. Blood cells include the erythrocytes—the red blood cells—as well as the leukocytes—the white blood cells—crucial components of the immune system.

This process of blood production, called hematopoiesis, occurs in the embryo and fetus in tissues such as the liver, thymus, and spleen, as well as the red marrow. After birth, the red marrow is primarily responsible for creating new blood, although tissues in the lymphatic system (see chapter 2) help in the production of some white blood cells. The ancestors of all of one's blood cells is a single population of primitive, permanent red bone marrow residents, the *stem cells*.

In the Beginning

Each of us began as a single cell. That potent cell formed in the upper reaches of the oviduct when any one of the millions of sperm cells, swirling about the delicate outer membrane of a ripe egg, penetrated it. Soon the cell settled down to its appointed business. Within hours the fertilized egg began to divide. Then the resulting two cells divided further into four, then eight, and so on, as the tiny embryo grew in size and complexity.

By twelve weeks after fertilization, long since attached to the warm protective lining of the uterus, the embryo had shaped itself into a minute human organism, now called the *fetus*, meaning "young one." This extraordinary development into a multicellular organism, with a maze of specialized cells and tissues—blood, muscle, nerves, glands—is by no means completed even at birth.

As we mature, a reservoir of cells remains hidden in our tissues, cells that are forever young and unspecialized: the stem cells, whose task it is to replenish cells that succumb to the wear and tear of life. For example, each of our red blood cells lives for about 120 days. Each second, about 2.5 million red cells in our circulatory system succumb to old age and are quickly replaced by fresh, new cells derived from stem cells in the red bone marrow. The white blood cells of the immune system, less numerous but equally vital, may survive for only a few days, and they, too, need replacing. As the stem cells respond to chemical cues and divide and differentiate into replacements, they replenish their own numbers as well, leaving an undiminished supply of stem cells, while their offspring head off into the bloodstream.

Going beyond the familiar formation of blood cells in the bone marrow, the intestinal lining, the epidermis, and (in males) the testes have long been recognized as sites where primitive stem cells continuously produce replacements for lost cells, while maintaining their own population. Stem cells also are present in very small concentrations in the circulating blood and in much greater numbers in the newborn's umbilical cord.

In April 1999, Mark Pittinger of Osiris Therapeutics in Baltimore, Maryland (www.osiristx.com), reported isolating stem cells from human bone marrow that were quite different from those that made blood cells. Unlike the marrow's stem cells, which supply the mature cells for the blood and immune system, these mesenchymal stem cells could be triggered in the laboratory to differentiate into fat, cartilage, and bone cells. Earlier, scientists had demonstrated that when bone marrow was injected into the blood of mice whose own marrow had been destroyed by radiation, some of the injected cells grew into replacements for a small fraction of the cells in bone, cartilage, lung, and several other tissues.

This means that the bone marrow contains a small subset of stem cells that are able to grow into tissues other than blood. The Osiris research went a step further in that they actually isolated individual stem cells from human bone marrow and grew each of them in the laboratory into colonies of more than a million identical stem cells. Then, by carefully manipulating the contents of the growth medium, they coaxed the stem cells into becoming bone, cartilage, or fat cells.

Others soon reported that human bone marrow, more precisely the mesenchymal stem cells, could metamorphose into liver cells. Likewise, researchers at Children's Hospital in Boston, Massachusetts (www.tch.harvard.edu), found that mouse bone marrow stem cells infused into mice weakened by muscular dystrophy not only generated new blood cells, but also migrated to the muscle and produced new, healthy muscle cells. It now appears likely that all repairable adult tissues probably harbor a population of stem cells.

In the late 1990's other researchers reported a series of extraordinary discoveries relating to stem cells in the nervous system. Stem cells were isolated from the forebrain of an aborted human fetus, grown in culture, and injected into mice brains, where they proceeded to develop into neurons and their support cells, the glia. In another experiment, mouse brain stem cells injected into a mouse partially healed the lesions of Parkinson's disease and multiple sclerosis, and when put into a mouse's bone marrow differentiated into bone marrow cells. In yet another case, the first neural stem cells from an adult animal were isolated from the ventricles lining rat brains as well as from rat spinal cords.

In early 2000, scientists from the University of Florida in Gainesville (www.ufl.edu) isolated stem cells from the pancreases of mice, got the cells to grow in laboratory culture, transplanted them into diabetic mice, and showed that the transplanted cells worked to produce insulin. The ability to remove stem cells from both animals and humans and to grow them in laboratory cultures has led to increased efforts to discover the genetic and chemical signals that lead the young, immature stem cells into mature, specialized cells.

Such knowledge could lead to a wide variety of unique and valuable medical treatments. Stem cells might be stimulated to convert into cells that could repair damaged tissues such as cartilage, heart, liver, kidney, skin, brain or spinal cord, leading to effective treatments for such disorders as diabetes, Parkinson's, muscular dystrophy, and spinal cord trauma. In the case of gene therapy, genes might be inserted into stem cells that could then be put into a person's bone marrow, where they would be a permanent source of the proteins made by the genes. Stem cells, once changed to either normal or even pathological adult cell types in culture, could be used for drug screening and to study the basics of the disease process.

The possible implications of these discoveries go far beyond our immediate interest, but there are several intriguing possibilities to keep in mind. Laboratory research on animals is already underway to try to perfect a way to insert stem cells primed to replace tissues lost to, for example, cancer, osteoporosis, injury, or destruction by RA. Not only may these stem cells replace tissues, they may carry with them genes that have been added to them in the laboratory, and once in place, the cells will produce their gene-made proteins, perhaps proteins that may protect against the disease that once affected those tissues.

This newfound ability to remove and use mesenchymal stem cells from adult tissues is also important because it avoids the controversy of using stem cells from human embryos. Since a series of research breakthroughs in 1998, human stem cell cultures now can be routinely grown from *embryonic stem cells* (*ES cells*) derived from the inner cell mass of the human embryo. The inner cell mass is a cluster of cells enclosed in the hollow ball of cells that forms when the fertilized egg undergoes repeated, rapid divisions. The inner cell mass is removed from human embryos that have been made in laboratory dishes in the process known as *in vitro* (literally, "in glass") fertilization. ES cells have the potential to differentiate into all types of specialized cells in the organism. These successes capped a seventeen-year race to isolate and culture human embryonic stem cells. The potential, as yet unrealized in a predictable fashion, to produce unlimited supplies of any cell or tissue in the body, was hailed as a revolution in science and medicine.

This led to objections from those who consider the resultant destruction of the human embryo as ethically unacceptable. A United States congressional ban in effect since 1995 had forbidden the use of federal funds for research that puts human embryos at risk. However, a January 19, 1999, decision by the Department of Health and Human Services (HHS) ruled that ES cells should be excluded from the ban because they, unlike whole embryos, lack the capacity to develop into full human organisms. That cleared the way for the NIH to provide funds for research on human ES cells from embryos obtained from a non-federally funded source.

In other words, federally funded research on ES cells can be carried out if the researchers use embryonic stem cells removed from embryos left over from clinics where fertilized eggs are implanted into women who could not otherwise become pregnant. The researchers are not allowed to create the embryos strictly for research purposes.

Stem cells for the possible regeneration of tissues relevant to RA, such as bone and cartilage, can be isolated from adults, too. However, research using ES cells continues in the search for insights into the intricate details of human development, as well as to supply cells that are potential sources of other tissues such as kidney, heart, and lungs.

There are a few human trials now using stem cells derived from adult tissues that are attempting to regenerate cartilage and bone lost to injury or disease. However, in people with RA, even when reparative regeneration is possible, it would not reverse or slow the relentless progress of the disease. In order to do that, stronger measures are needed.

STEM CELLS TO THE RESCUE

Bone marrow transplants (*BMTs*) are sometimes performed when a person's bone marrow is so damaged or diseased that it cannot function normally. High-dose chemotherapy and/or radiation therapy, accompanied by BMT, is a standard treatment for some malignancies, such as various forms of leukemia, and is under study in clinical trials for other conditions, including ovarian and lung cancers. A transplant in which the marrow comes from another person is called an *allogeneic* transplant. If, as may often be the case, the bone marrow is taken from a donor and then given back later to that same donor, the procedure is called an *autologous* transplant.

In the allogeneic transplant, because the immune system of the recipient will, as we have pointed out, reject any foreign cells, including bone marrow, a donor must be found whose marrow is as compatible as possible with the recipient. Although an unrelated person can be a donor, an identical twin is ideal (in which case it would be a *syngeneic* transplant) or a compatible sibling. There is a one in four chance that any brother or sister will be an acceptable match. The real point of bone marrow transplants is to supply the recipient with new stem cells, which are distributed throughout the rich red marrow.

During marrow collection, general or spinal anesthesia is used, and about a quart of marrow is removed from the hip bones of the donor with a sterile needle. In an allogeneic transplant the marrow is processed and given to the recipient within several hours. For an autologous transplant, the marrow is frozen to use at a later date.

The first successful bone marrow transplant was performed in 1968. Two children were cured of severe immune system deficiencies. A more efficient way to give a higher concentration of stem cells was initiated in 1984 in the form of the peripheral blood stem cell transplant (PBSCT). Most stem cells live in the bone marrow, but smaller numbers also circulate in the bloodstream, at a concentration about ten thousand times less than that in the marrow. Because of that, a much greater volume of blood has to be processed in order to get the necessary number of stem cells. This is done using a machine that separates the various types of blood cells so that only the fraction of blood containing the stem cells is retained and the rest of the blood is returned to the donor.

The blood is collected through a tube placed in a large vein. The blood flows through the cell separator, where the stem cells are retained and the rest returns directly to the donor. This *apheresis* takes about two to four hours, and several sessions are usually needed.

The bone marrow or, more commonly, the stem cell preparation, is given to the recipient as a blood transfusion. Once the cells pass into the bloodstream, the stem cells find their way back to the bones, settle down, and in a few weeks the stem cells will begin to manufacture new red and white cells. It may take considerably longer, however, for the immune system to recover.

While marrow and stem cell transplants have become in one sense a "routine" procedure, they can be a difficult, traumatic experience for the recipient, who is already under stress from disease and faces an uncertain future. Because healthy bone marrow must answer the constant demand for new red and white blood cells, any interruption in this life-support system has serious consequences, and even though the transplant usually "takes," there remains a long period of gradual recovery. During that period a low white cell count puts the recipient in danger of life-threatening infections; moreover, the resulting paucity of red cells leads to severe anemia with its accompanying weakness, headache, and lack of energy. Red blood cell transfusions may then be needed. After a marrow transplant organ dysfunctions can develop in the liver, kidneys, or lungs. Given all that the recipient goes through, the psychological stress is as troubling as the physical, as he or she fights distress, anxiety, or depression.

Despite all the difficulties that may accompany a bone marrow/stem cell transplant, not to mention the formidable expense, these rich infusions of fresh cells may sometimes save a life. In aplastic anemia, for example, a disease in which the bone marrow stops working, transplants have a cure rate of 80 percent (www.aamds-international.org). This leads us to an important question. *Might it be possible to follow this example and get rid of RA by replacing the old marrow with new? Could one, in effect, "reboot" the bone marrow and make a fresh, new immune system, leaving RA as only a bad memory?*

✚ ✚ ✚

In 1981, a fifty-two-year-old woman with severe RA suffered damage to her bone marrow after receiving injections of gold salts in an effort to relieve her arthritis symptoms. She instead ended up with severe anemia. She was then given a transfusion of bone marrow donated by her healthy brother in the hopes that it might restore her ability to again make blood cells. Before she received the new marrow, her doctors administered powerful drugs followed by total body irradiation in order to suppress her immune system so that she would not reject the marrow transplant.

After recovering from the grueling procedure, she was discharged from the hospital on only a low dose of prednisone, a common steroid medication (see chapter 7). For two years, she experienced complete remission from her RA symptoms. Over the next eleven years, many of her symptoms returned nevertheless, with progressive joint damage and deformity, but with less pain and tenderness. This long-term follow-up of the 1981 transplant contained a detailed analysis, including X-rays, and was done a very long time after the transplant as compared to the few other studies.

By 1997, of the seven reported cases of people with RA who had undergone a bone marrow transplant for severe anemia, three had died of transplant-related complications within months of the procedure, one was alive and free of arthritis two years post-BMT, and another had some residual joint pain after three years. A sixth person was free of pain, without medication, six years post-BMT, while the seventh was reported in complete remission after six years.

In addition to offering another reminder of the possibility of fatal consequences after a marrow transplant, these cases raised some important questions. When symptoms returned, was this the "original" RA coming back after temporary suppression or the development of a "new" RA from the donor's immune cells, activated by an antigen in the recipient? Perhaps bone marrow-derived immune system cells did not play a role in the redevelopment of RA?

Whatever the explanation, these experiences and others showed that despite initial hopes that bone marrow transplants might "cure" RA, it appeared that RA could recur and even continue to worsen years after the transplant. Attention turned to refinements of marrow transplants, particularly regarding the source of the marrow. In the cases cited above the transplant was allogeneic, that is, from someone other than the recipient.

Investigations began in 1996 on perfecting techniques for removing stem cells from the marrow of a person with an autoimmune disease such as RA or lupus, with the intention of giving those cells back to the same person after eradicating the rest of the marrow—hoping for a fresh start.

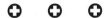

By late 1996, physicians at Sir Charles Gairdner Hospital, Nedlands, Western Australia (www.scgh.health.wa.gov.au), had tried every available treatment for a forty-six-year-old man with severe RA, to no avail. By then, seven years after coming down with the disease, he had had both hips replaced, could move about only in an electric wheelchair, and in the previous year had spent only thirty days out of the hospital. After clearance by the institutional ethics committee, researchers—headed by David J. L. Joske—began the careful, slow process of removing stem cells from his bloodstream. They first administered special drugs, including granulocyte colony-stimulating factor (G-CSF). These chemicals flushed stem cells hidden in his bone marrow into his blood, thus greatly enriching the stem cell concentration. Three weeks later, after a drug regime to suppress his own bone marrow, they gave him back his concentrated stem cells. In a few weeks his joint symptoms had abated noticeably. At six months, he walked more than a mile with ease. *He was the first person to have been specifically treated for RA with an autologous (his own) stem cell transplant—and with remarkable results.*

In 1997, in the Hospital at the Free University of Brussels, Brussels, Belgium (www.vub.ac.be), researchers received permission from the hospital ethics committee to perform an autologous stem cell transplant on a twenty-two-year-old woman whose RA was unaffected by any available medications. As in the first case described above, her stem cells were removed by apheresis, using the machine that separates out various types of blood cells, after she was given drugs to move stem cells into her blood from her bone marrow. In an additional step, her blood was treated with the Isolex 300i, developed by Nexell Therapeutics, Irvine, California (www.nexellinc.com).

This ingenious device exposes the blood to special protein antibodies that attach only to the stem cells. Microscopic metal beads then grab onto the antibodies, and the stem cell–antibody-bead sandwiches are held by a magnetic field, thus effectively separating them from the other marrow cells. In a similar fashion the T cells, long implicated in the inflammatory and destructive pathways in RA, are pulled out of the mix and discarded. The magnetic field is turned off, the antibodies and beads stripped from the stem cells, leaving a mix of T cell–depleted, richly concentrated stem cells. After the young woman's bone marrow was depleted with powerful chemicals, the stem cells were returned to her. Ten months later, she was judged to be free of her RA, and needed no medications. As of mid-2000 she was still in the same happy state.

✪   ✪   ✪

In 1998, a team of researchers headed by Richard K. Burt of Northwestern Memorial Hospital (www.nmh.org) and Northwestern University in Chicago, Illinois, reported the results of autologous stem cell transplants on ten people—six with multiple sclerosis, two with lupus, and two with RA. After a procedure quite similar to the Belgium technique described above, all those subjects with multiple sclerosis, despite the fact that they had rapidly progressive disease before the transplant, showed no signs of disease progression after checkups ranging from five to seventeen months.

Those with lupus fared as well, showing no evidence of active disease up to one year post-transplant. And the people with RA? The first, a forty-six-year-old woman, showed considerable improvement even after twelve months; while the second, a forty-two-year-old -woman, showed less, but still welcome relief. Both had fewer swollen joints, were able to go about their daily activities with less discomfort and reduced medications. One year later, Dr. Burt and many of the same associates reported on another series of stem cell transplants in four people with RA. In this series, two obtained significant relief for nine and twenty months post-treatment, while the others did not enjoy any sustained response.

✛   ✛   ✛

A small percentage of children with severe juvenile rheumatoid arthritis do not respond to even powerful medications. Many of these children suffer severe joint destruction and adverse effects from attempts to limit the progress of their disease with such drugs. In February 1999, a report was published on a clinical trial at the University Hospital for Children, Utrecht, the Netherlands (www.ziekenhuis.nl). Four youngsters, aged six to eleven years, became the first children to undergo stem cell transplants for their chronic, disabling arthritis.

Nico Wulffraat and his colleagues used marrow from the children's hips, rather than from circulating blood. They carefully purged the marrow of T cells, and treated the children with anti–T cell antibodies and anti–T cell drugs, which were followed by total body irradiation to wipe out the remaining marrow and immune cells. They then infused the purged marrow back into the children in the hope that the stem cells would create a new immune system with new T cells that would fight infections but not attack the children's joints.

After six to eighteen months, all four children, off all medications, showed a marked decrease in joint swelling, pain, and morning stiffness. The researchers were careful to point out in their February 1999 report that ". . . the actual follow-up is too short, however, to conclude that these children are completely cured of their disease."

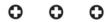

In Ottawa, Canada, a twenty-three-year-old woman, suffering from juvenile rheumatoid arthritis that had attacked virtually every joint in her body, had not gotten any relief despite having used every available medication. She became the first person in Canada to receive a stem cell transplant for RA. Doctors at the Ottawa Hospital (www.ogh.on.ca) harvested stem cells from her blood, cleansed them of T cells, and, after obliterating her bone marrow, gave her back the concentrated, purified stem cells in March 1999. A year later she was leading a normal life, virtually free of the pain that she had endured for years. Her blood tests, including those that reflect inflammation, were, according to her physician, Dr. Robert McKendry, "absolutely normal." He points out, however, that she was not in total remission from her disease because she still had several tender joints.

The Past Leading to the Future

The notion of wiping out a person's bone marrow, thereby removing her capacity to make blood cells, and then rebuilding new marrow by transfusions of stem cells in order to treat severe autoimmune disease was first proposed in 1993. Extensive trials with experimental animals, usually mice, had shown that this radical procedure suggested some promise of refurbishing the disease-ravaged immune systems of these experimental animals. In humans, there have been very intriguing results accompanying a series of bone marrow transplants in people who were being treated for diseases such as leukemia and who also happened to have RA. The transplants gave some relief from the arthritis as well as the leukemia. These experiences convinced scientists to move ahead with the idea to clinical trials.

By mid-2000, about 350 people had undergone some variation of stem cell transplants for autoimmune diseases. The procedures were almost all autologous transplants. In other words, subjects got back their own stem cells, which had been collected from them earlier. In most cases, high doses of drugs and/or growth factors first were employed to drive stem cells from the subject's marrow into the bloodstream. The blood, circulated through an apheresis device before being returned to the subject, was often treated to increase the stem cell concentration and/or to remove T or B cells.

The person usually returned about one month later. Drugs and/or radiation were administered to the individual to wipe out his bone marrow, and the rich stem cell mix was infused intravenously. Within ten to twelve days the stem cells had settled down in the hollow interior of the bones and, as though oblivious to their foreign travels, were dividing rapidly and making life-sustaining supplies of new blood cells.

Lest this description appear to be describing a benign and almost routine procedure, note that autologous stem cell transplantation for autoimmune disease—getting back one's own stem cells after marrow destruction—carries with it an overall mortality (death) rate of 8 to 9 percent, and for RA, about 2.5 percent.

In these kinds of clinical trials, only people who have a significant risk to their lives or to their vital organs are chosen for a transplant—with their informed consent, of course. By mid-2000 there were data on 275 transplants done at sixty-four centers from twenty countries. This information is located in a database in Basel, Switzerland, under the auspices of the European Group for Blood and Marrow Transplantation (EBMT; gildor.conexis.es), working in cooperation with the European League Against Rheumatism (EULAR; www.eular.org) International Autoimmune Disease Stem Cell Project.

Also, about fifty cases are registered in the Milwaukee-based International Bone Marrow Transplant Registry (IBMTR; www.ibmtr.org), and almost fifty unregistered transplants have been published. This means, as noted earlier, that almost 350 people with severe autoimmune disease have undergone this procedure, at least 40 of whom have had RA or JRA. The welcome international coordination has allowed more precise definitions of which individuals are best suited for inclusion in these trials.

In seeking a cure for RA and other autoimmune diseases through transplants, there are certain challenges to be considered. One is that through this drastic procedure we will literally have to replace all the immune system cells that react against the person's own tissues, like the T cells and B cells, and replace them with healthy, nonreactive cells. In theory, that would best be accomplished by giving someone stem cells from another compatible person; in other words, an allogeneic transplant. Then, at least ideally, the new cells from the donor would become a new immune system, and wipe out any remaining self-reactive cells left over in the recipient.

However, the dangers of more serious side effects and deaths of the recipients of allogeneic transplants than from autologous have favored the use of the latter. If the person's stem cells themselves are normal, and if rebuilding an immune system with these stem cells after wiping out the bone marrow removes any trace of cells that can react against that person's own tissues and cause RA to reignite, then a real cure is possible. On the other hand, if trouble-causing cells remain within the marrow, or are put back into the person along with the treated stem cells, then a relapse of RA may be inevitable.

As we look over all the trials reported so far, certain generalities begin to emerge, even at this early date. As of early 2000, for RA, the condition of fourteen of the thirty-five subjects evaluated three months after transplant was reported as "better," while six were "worse." For JRA, sixteen of twenty-five were "better" and only one was "worse." Also, removing T cells before returning the stem cells seemed to make little difference in this rate. The jury is still out on the question of whether or not a cure for RA is possible using stem cell transplants.

Between 1995 and 2000 there were numerous meetings and conferences among the growing number of researchers intent on coordinating and improving their efforts to maximize stem cell transplantation in the fight against autoimmune disease. Some agreements were reached on parameters for certain clinical trials, including those for multiple sclerosis and JRA, and posted on the Web site of the EBMT (gildor.conexis.es/ebmt), while RA trial design remained under discussion. In the United States, fifteen centers have formed the National Collaborative Study for Stem Cell Transplant for Autoimmune Disease, known as the Seattle Protocols Group.

With so many diverse institutions now working toward a common goal, it is essential to collect and centralize the facts and figures relating to the methods used and the results achieved. After several years of international collaboration among EULAR, EMBT, IBMTR, the American College of Rheumatology, the National Institutes of Health (NIH), and other groups dedicated to eradicating these diseases, standardized data forms have been agreed on for several autoimmune diseases, including RA and JRA. They are available on the Web for registered specialists. In October 2000, an international meeting took place in Basel, Switzerland, to review all the data and plan trials.

✪   ✪   ✪

What are we to conclude from all this? Stem cell transplants to treat severe RA, as well as other autoimmune diseases such as lupus and multiple sclerosis, are being performed worldwide in increasing numbers and with various modifications, in the hope of optimizing the results and reducing the danger. International conferences continue to be held and other forms of widespread cooperation among researchers are accelerating. Not only will stem cell transplant methods improve, but careful study of the recovery of the immune system after stem cell transplants may uncover important details about the inner workings of RA.

A stem cell transplant, still only in the experimental stage, should be seen realistically as a very expensive, risky process. It may not, in fact, lead to a cure. But for the growing number of people for whom this procedure has meant a new life, it has been nothing short of a miracle.

What about the vast majority of people with RA for whom a miracle is not in the cards? There are, in fact, a number of medications that have been available for a long time, targeting various sites within the immune system, that can help manage the pain and suffering that so often accompanies RA. In addition to these "traditional" pharmaceuticals, there is a brand-new family of medicines available that has recently revolutionized the approach to RA treatment. Let's look inside the rheumatology medicine cabinet to better understand what relief is available right now.

CHAPTER 7

Inside the
Medicine Cabinet

D r. William Oliver, a celebrated mid-eighteenth-century English physician and founder of a popular rheumatic hospital in Bath, England, wrote in 1751 that rheumatoid arthritis was "... certain a most stubborn distemper, and has baffled all the professors of Physick that ever have appeared in the World. The cause lies too deep for any Medicine or Method yet known to come to the bottom of it."

The frustrating search for the cause of RA and for effective means of relief from pain and disability had undoubtedly gone on for centuries before Dr. Oliver made his pessimistic analysis. While it is difficult to pick out as certain which important figures in history were burdened with RA, it seems probable that they included such notables as Christopher Columbus (1451–1506) and Mary, Queen of Scots (1542–1587). By 1500, Columbus's joints were constantly swollen and aching to the point that he had to be tied to the mast in order not to be swept overboard. As for Mary, by 1587 she could barely walk, and had to be supported by two assistants as she limped to her unfortunate end on the scaffold. Nearer to our own time, President James Madison wrote in 1832, "... my fingers make smaller letters, and my feet make smaller steps, but my heart survives." Madison "treated" his RA by periodic fasts. He had to retain a special secretary to keep track of the flood of "cures" that fellow sufferers sent to him from all parts of the world.

The plight of the rich and famous would probably not have inspired the ample diversity of often bizarre therapies tried out over the centuries, were it not for the fact that RA has touched the lives of so many millions of ordinary people as well. Inhibited by an ignorance of even the most basic understanding of the body's functions, and faced with an often painful and debilitating disease, it is understandable that people devised what would seem to us outlandish attempts to get some relief.

The Roman physician Scribonius Largus liked to take his clients to the beach at Ostia, near Rome, and place their feet on a large torpedo fish, which responded by giving them a nasty jolt of electricity. He insisted that this led to several permanent cures, although one could understand why his patients might not want to report any further complaints.

The "home remedy" approach to RA continued unabated well into the twentieth century (and continues today). David Cantor, writing in 1992 on medical innovations in historical perspective, describes 1949 as featuring a "bumper crop of rheumatism cures and treatments." Among the most fanciful were the use of bee stings, an "adrenaline vanishing cream," a South African molasses treatment, and, from Sweden, a hothouse regimen. The Belgians boasted a therapy of copper salts, while in the United States, Boston doctors inserted nylon strips into knee joints, and in Miami, the wolf fat cure was highly touted.

Cantor chose the year 1949 not because of the above "cures," but because of another announcement hidden in the welter of claims. This one said that a derivative of ox blood might cure RA, "although 200,000 cattle would be needed to produce a mere 2700 grams of the substance." This supposedly miraculous substance, in what sounds like just another outlandish notion was *cortisone*, which would revolutionize the treatment of inflammation, although not without severe limitations, as we will see shortly.

✚ ✚ ✚

It was really only in the last half of the twentieth century that the treatment of RA began to emphasize the "empirical" approach; that is, one based on experimentation and observation rather than on theory. That is simply because only in recent years have researchers begun to uncover the details of the basic processes of the disease, which are buried in the complexities of the human immune system. In fact, we have made major strides only in the last few years in the understanding of what is happening in the cells and tissues of people with RA.

In 1996, a statement in the "Guidelines for the Management of RA" published by the American College of Rheumatology (ACR) said that, "Until the cause of rheumatoid arthritis (RA) is further elucidated, a successful prevention or repair of such tissue destruction remains elusive." Elusive though it may be, the advances in our understanding of what lies behind the inflammation and tissue destruction in RA continues at a rapid pace. In November 1998, Bevra Hahn, president of the ACR, could tell the audience at the ACR National Scientific Meeting : "This is an exciting time for rheumatology . . . after years of research, we now have multiple options for our patients." American rheumatology has come a long way since June 1934, when the new American Rheumatism Association (which would eventually evolve into the ACR in 1988) met in Cleveland to hear a mere eleven research papers.

Early in the twenty-first century the optimism for finding newer and more effective RA medications continues as a contingent of innovative and unique RA pharmaceuticals, based on a growing understanding of the chemical messages used by the immune system, becomes available to physicians. As we describe these as well as the more traditional but often useful drugs, it is important to keep several things in perspective.

We do not yet have therapies that we know will cure RA or predictably stop the progression of the disease in its tracks. Certainly there are many instances in which people with RA achieve dramatic relief through medications prescribed by their physicians. There are brand-new medications, and more soon to arrive, that will suppress symptoms and sometimes halt disease progression, for which physicians and people with RA alike are most grateful. We will describe those medications as well as discuss the exciting possibilities opened up by recent research. And yet we have to be straightforward and admit that we still do not fully understand what causes or perpetuates RA. That means that, despite the fact that while we are a very long way from the days when a physician's treatments fared no better than folk medicine, David Fox, a prominent American rheumatologist, could still write in 2000 that the "treatment of RA remains insufficiently effective and distressingly toxic for many patients."

In the current treatment of a person with RA, while the ultimate hope is to induce a complete remission, which occurs only rarely, the major goals are: to reduce pain and discomfort, to reduce the probability of irreversible joint damage, to maintain function for the essential activities of daily living, and to maximize the person's quality of life. Within the last few years, the possibility of attaining those goals is more realistic than it ever has been. While a well-rounded program of RA treatment certainly goes beyond the use of pharmaceuticals to include the important components of exercise, physical therapy, and adequate and timely rest, our emphasis here is on the available and soon-to-be-available medications.

Although there certainly is general agreement about strategies that are used in employing medications as part of a program to control RA, there is by no means a single, universally applied approach. There are several reasons for this. In the first place, RA is a tricky disease to manage because of the waxing and waning nature of the symptoms. About 80 percent of people with RA show a cyclical pattern of symptoms, that is, one in which they experience periodic *remission,* in which the disease appears to "slow down." These remissions, which may last up to a year, are followed by a "speeding up" of the symptoms, called a *flare.* Another 10 percent have an acute episode and then enter a permanent remission. About 10 percent experience a debilitating progression that leads to severe bone erosion and permanent disability.

Also, not only do people differ, often unpredictably, in the course of their disease, but they also vary in their responses to medications. Despite the fact that certain medications may be quite effective for particular individuals, as a rule of thumb all of the medications traditionally used for RA have little effect for about 25 percent of people who try them.

In the final analysis, the choice of medications requires that a number of factors be considered by the physician (ideally, a rheumatologist) and the individual with RA. Entering into how best to decide on a treatment regimen together are: the stage of the disease and its anticipated course, the time needed for response to the medications, the cost, an allergy to a drug's component or potential for interaction with another drug, the physician's experience with similar situations, and her knowledge and interpretation of the latest research findings. Even though a particular drug may be very effective in controlling a person's pain and inflammation, those benefits must always be balanced by the chance of unwanted side effects, a complication that can differ widely among individuals.

With that in mind, let's review the more traditional means

of treating RA and see how they are now evolving in light of more recent discoveries. While these "standard" methods of treatment often have been effective in reducing pain and inflammation for many people, they were not always instituted based on a sound knowledge of their exact effects on the cellular, chemical pathways of the disease. After all, those pathways were not well known at the time.

Our increasing understanding of the chemical messages sent and received by cells during inflammation and their effects in the tissues of people with RA, which has led to the formulation of new and innovative therapies (see chapters 8 and 9), has also given us new insights into how more traditional medications work. It also helps to suggest ways to improve their effectiveness. Moreover, between 1995 and 2000, there was a major move toward combination therapy. This means that RA treatment for many began to feature new combinations of the traditional medications described below as well as the addition of newer drugs not available until the late 1990s. We will look at this new approach after we describe the traditional medications.

THE BASIC MEDICINE CABINET

Traditional treatment for RA has employed three classes of drugs: *NSAIDs*—nonsteroidal anti-inflammatory drugs (pronounced "en-seds"); *DMARDs*—disease-modifying antirheumatic drugs (pronounced "dee-mards"); and *steroids*—often called corticosteroids or glucocorticosteroids.

Let's look at the major features of each of these relative to RA. You have probably seen those pages of fine print enclosed in medication packages that describe every bit of information you could possibly want about a particular drug, from its possible side effects to its chemical formula. Our look at RA medications will emphasize the most immediately relevant facts. Comprehensive, easy-to-follow information about drugs can be found, among many other sites, at www.mayohealth.org and www.pharminfo.com. We'll use the generic or common name of the drugs, as well as the brand names, as they are designated in the United States. These same medications are sold internationally under a variety of other brand names.

NSAIDs

This rather complicated name, "nonsteroidal anti-inflammatory drugs," means simply that these NSAIDs retard inflammation and they are not steroids, which are powerful hormones also used to treat RA. NSAIDs, which include aspirin, as well as about twenty other drugs mostly available only by prescription, have been used for many years to alleviate pain and inflammation caused by a variety of ailments. They are the most widely prescribed class of drugs in all of medicine. NSAIDs have been the most commonly used antiarthritis agents since the Bayer Company in Germany formulated the pain reliever acetylsalicylic acid, or aspirin, in the late 1800s. The first modern NSAID, indomethacin (Indocin) came on the scene in 1965. Almost 300 million people take NSAIDs daily, about one-third of whom have RA or osteoarthritis. In 1984 ibuprofen joined aspirin as an over-the-counter NSAID. Popular brand names are Advil, Motrin, and Nuprin. This was later joined by naproxen sodium (Naprosyn) and ketoprofen (Orudis).

Most other varieties of NSAIDs are available only by prescription. While aspirin remains an economical, effective choice, the amounts needed in RA require multiple daily doses and may lead to serious stomach irritation and even ulceration or decreased kidney function. While there are safer, chemically modified forms of aspirin, and rheumatologists often prescribe them first, aspirin in its various forms has largely been replaced by other NSAIDs as the initial choice of drug therapy for RA. Using these NSAIDs requires taking fewer pills and tends to be less irritating, but side effects can still occur, including stomach upset or ulceration. In fact, there is an annual incidence of 1 to 2 percent of ulcers and bleeding in people with RA who are long-term users of NSAIDs.

Unfortunately, serious gastrointestinal complications among NSAID users usually occur suddenly, with little or no warning. In 1997 more than one hundred thousand people in the United States were hospitalized for gastrointestinal problems connected to NSAID use. For people taking NSAIDs who are considered at greater risk—for example, those with a history of ulcers—there are medications to help prevent these complications, such as misoprostol (Cytotec). People with normal kidney function are at low risk of NSAID-induced kidney damage, but people who have decreased kidney function because of, for example, congestive heart failure, and the elderly are at a greater risk. Also, to be on the safe side, most physicians do not consider NSAIDs to be safe for use during pregnancy.

Paradoxically, the very reason that these NSAIDs may produce unwanted side effects is the same reason that they are so effective against pain and inflammation. When these medications, usually taken orally, are carried by the blood into the body's tissues, NSAIDs work by blocking the activity of a common enzyme, abbreviated as *COX*. This enzyme is responsible for making *prostaglandins*. There are many different types of prostaglandins. Some contribute to the pain and inflammation of RA, but other kind of prostaglandins are beneficial. For example, they help the stomach resist ulcer formation.

Only in the late 1970s did we realize that inhibition of the COX enzyme was the molecular mechanism behind the relief that had been achieved with aspirin for almost one hundred years. The English scientist Sir John Vane received the Nobel Prize in Physiology or Medicine in 1982 for this discovery, and his insight led to the formulation of many other NSAIDs that could act in the same way.

The prostaglandins, among their many effects in the body, are major contributors to pain and inflammation. In RA the inflamed synovial tissues lining the joints use a variety of different cells to make large quantities of prostaglandins, in response to those chemical messages that we have mentioned often, TNF-alpha and IL-1. It is no wonder that cutting down on prostaglandin production brings some relief. While some studies have shown that NSAIDs can actually slow the progression of RA to some degree in certain people, for most, regrettably, neither aspirin nor any of the other NSAIDs can alter the course of RA or prevent joint destruction in the long run.

In the early 1990s, further research on the COX enzyme revealed that there are actually two distinct forms of the enzyme, *COX-1* and *COX-2*. The COX-1 form makes the kinds of prostaglandins that are always found in many tissues such as the stomach and the kidneys, and helps to keep them healthy and free from irritation. For example, in the stomach these prostaglandins stimulate mucus and bicarbonate secretion (the active ingredient in Alka-Seltzer). In the kidneys, they help to maintain a healthy blood flow and stimulate salt excretion.

On the other hand, it is the COX-2 type that makes the prostaglandins that are found at sites of tissue inflammation. It turns out that typical NSAIDs slow down the activity of both forms of the enzyme. One the one hand, they can suppress inflammation by inhibiting COX-2, but simultaneously turn off the helpful COX-1—a mixed blessing.

Given this important insight, it makes sense that scientists turned to creating drugs that would specifically block COX-2, and therefore suppress inflammation, while sparing COX-1, the helpful enzyme. This research soon resulted in the late 1990s in a revolution in the world of NSAIDs—new forms now available that selectively inhibit COX-2 and have far fewer undesirable side effects (see chapter 8).

Neither the newer or the older NSAIDs can be depended upon to stop the long-term progress of RA. Research has not shown any significant differences in efficacy among the various forms of NSAIDs. As is true with so many medications, response to NSAIDs differs greatly among individuals, and NSAIDs can and do give some relief from pain and swelling. Pain relief is generally quick, while the anti-inflammatory effect may not take hold for four to six weeks. While NSAID benefits fall far short of a cure, and they have limitations, they have lightened the burden of RA for millions through their use.

DMARDs

DMARDs are the "disease-modifying antirheumatic drugs." They are also often referred to as *SAARDs*, meaning "slow-acting antirheumatic drugs," or as second-line agents. The description "disease-modifying" is not necessarily an accurate portrayal of our current understanding and use of these medications. Studies continue as to what extent DMARDs actually do alter the course of RA and improve long-term outcomes. There is evidence that there can be at least a 30 percent reduction in long-term disability with consistent DMARD use. The "slow-acting" description may not only signify that they may take weeks or months to work, but also reflect a low effectiveness on inflamed joints. The term "second-line," meaning the drugs of choice after using NSAIDs, is applied less and less as these drugs are prescribed earlier than in the recent past. Be that as it may, it is important to recognize that DMARDs do have an effect on RA that is more delayed and different than NSAIDs. For many people they can be quite effective and bring about a significant improvement in symptoms.

One of the techniques for judging whether or not particular DMARDs can control the damage that RA can cause in the joints is to take X-rays, usually of the hands, wrists, or feet, early in the disease and then over a period of time. Increase in joint damage is not always easy to assess and ideally should be done over an extended period of time. Studies indicate that DMARDs, particularly methotrexate and sulfasalazine, discussed below, can retard the rate of progression of damage in the joints.

Because RA can lead to irreversible joint and bone damage, the more conservative approach to initial use of DMARDs is changing. In 1996, the ACR wrote a new set of guidelines for the management of RA. The recommendations underline that all people "whose RA remains active despite adequate treatment with NSAIDs are candidates for DMARD therapy." They recommend that this addition of DMARDs not be delayed beyond three months. They point out that people who have active RA marked by pain and swelling in multiple joints and who have rheumatoid factor in their blood stand a greater than 70 percent chance of developing joint damage or bone erosions within two years of the beginning of the disease. By 2000, as we point out at the conclusion of this chapter, DMARDs in various combinations were increasingly being used as soon as the RA was diagnosed.

That is why current treatment of RA tends to feature early, aggressive treatment, which means the use of DMARDs, often in conjunction with NSAIDs. According to the guidelines, "the goal of treatment is to intervene in the disease *before* joints are damaged."

The DMARDs described below share many characteristics. It may be months before any significant response to their use is evident, and each has a potential for toxic effects that requires careful monitoring. Because people have their own specific reactions to medications, it is impossible to predict exactly which DMARD is best for a particular individual, but up to two-thirds of people do show some positive response to DMARDs.

There are a number of factors that enter into the decision as to which DMARD to prescribe. The physician needs to consider the general health of the person, the severity of her RA, the time of expected benefit, the cost, the possible side effects, and the kind of monitoring needed to keep an eye out for adverse reactions. There is no "best" initial DMARD for people with RA, but certain generalities are noted below. It is clear that while individual DMARDs pose different levels of risk to the fetus, DMARDs in general are not recommended for use during pregnancy.

Like aspirin, DMARDs came into use years before we had an idea of how they actually worked. As a matter of fact, we still do not have a complete picture of exactly how each of them modifies the inner workings of our cells. As that picture becomes clearer through research, we can modify and improve on these "standard" medications, and design others that refine their beneficial effects and reduce their toxicity.

Many people with RA do not get sufficient relief from taking a single DMARD. The tendency in the last few years has been to try various combinations based on a series of ongoing clinical studies. The latest recommendations for combinations are discussed below, at the end of the description of the common DMARDs.

Methotrexate

Methotrexate (Rheumatrex) has been used for many years to treat cancers such as leukemia and lymphoma. Over the last thirty years its uses expanded to encompass many rheumatic diseases, as well as other illnesses such as asthma. Methotrexate, often referred to simply as MTX, was approved by the FDA in 1988 for use against RA. It has become the preferred drug in the arsenal of DMARDs for the management of that disease.

"Preferred" means that it has come to be the drug of choice for those people with the more severe form of RA, for example, those who have bone erosions, or are likely to develop them. MTX, if effective, usually begins to have some beneficial effects within several weeks of starting therapy. The typical, once-weekly oral dose is convenient and relatively inexpensive (about $600 per year), although for children the dosage is higher and is often given by injection.

Although many people can experience dramatic relief from the pain, swelling, and stiffness of inflammation through the use of MTX, it is uncommon to attain a complete remission of symptoms. If the drug is discontinued, inflammation usually reappears within weeks. The fire of RA is not put out, it just smolders. One is then faced with using MTX on a long-term basis. MTX and steroids (described later in this chapter) are the only DMARDs that are continued by more than 50 percent of people with RA versus 20 percent for the other DMARDs. A survey of U.S. rheumatologists published in 1998 rated MTX as the most effective DMARD after one and four years of treatment. Ninety percent of respondents judged it as excellent after one year, and 65 percent after four years.

As with any potent drug, there are possible side effects that warrant careful monitoring. The main concern is with potential damage to the liver, so that physicians need to be made aware of risk factors such as obesity, diabetes, alcohol intake, or a history of hepatitis B or C, all of which put additional stress on the liver. However, severe liver damage to people receiving long-term MTX is low, and there are sensitive blood tests for monitoring liver function.

As is typical with most DMARDs, we do not have a clear picture of how MTX interferes with RA. We have known for years that once it gets inside human cells it blocks the production of folic acid, a common vitamin. This interferes with a number of chemical pathways in cells. That is why when MTX is used for cancer, at far higher doses than are given for RA, there is a halt in the production of DNA, resulting in the death of cells, especially in the rapidly dividing cells of cancerous tumors.

A series of research studies in the 1990s have given us new insights into how MTX works. One of the pathways that it blocks results in the release of an anti-inflammatory chemical from cells that have taken in the MTX. This chemical fits right into the picture of inflammation that we described earlier, because it plugs up receptors on cells in inflamed joints and slows down the activity of those infamous inflammatory chemicals, TNF- alpha and IL-1.

Understanding these kinds of details is of more than just academic interest to scientists and pharmaceutical companies. It can lead to the creation of nontoxic RA medications that are aimed precisely at those receptor sites. In addition to the laudable goal of relieving the suffering of the approximately 50 million people now afflicted with RA, the fact that in 1999, sales of RA therapies worldwide totaled almost $1.5 billion has lent a strong impetus to this kind of research and development.

Hydroxychloroquine

It may seem a bit strange that hydroxychloroquine, which is also prescribed for acute malaria attacks, should have been called into service against RA. It is just another good example of how, over the years, medications that have been directed at other medical problems, and were observed to give some relief from RA, were added to the medicine cabinet without really understanding how they achieve their beneficial effects.

Quinine, a natural substance derived from the bark of a

tropical tree, has been an effective antimalarial for centuries. A derivative of quinine, Quinacrine (Atabrine), also used against malaria (as well as intestinal parasites), was first used in the 1950s to treat RA. Now physicians usually prescribe the newer hydroxychloroquine sulfate (Plaquenil) for people with early, less aggressive, mild to moderate RA, who usually lack the rheumatoid factor in their blood. Almost half the people in this category who take Plaquenil achieve some relief from symptoms within two to six months. If not, its use is usually discontinued.

A regimen of one or two inexpensive tablets daily and its low toxicity make this a convenient choice. Despite the relatively low incidence of adverse effects, including skin rash and stomach pain, there remains the concern over the very slight possibility of severe damage to the retina of the eye. Therefore, regular eye exams are always recommended for those taking this DMARD.

There is some evidence that this drug may make the internal contents of cells more alkaline, and retard their release of cytokines, those chemical messengers that perpetuate inflammation. Whatever the case, the effectiveness of this medication in a relatively small group of people underlines again the variable nature of the disease processes underlying RA. What works for some will not work for others.

Sulfasalazine

Back in 1939, before the age of antibiotics, the hunch that RA might be caused by a bacterial infection led Professor Nanna Svartz in Stockholm, Sweden, to combine salicylic acid, a component of aspirin, with various antibacterial chemicals called sulfonamides. One of the combinations, sulfasalazine, seemed to have some effect on RA. It has been used for decades, more commonly in Europe, and over the last few years has been prescribed more frequently in the United States after newer studies showed positive results. Sulfasalazine (Azulfidine), now available in coated tablets to minimize stomach irritation, is also given in the treatment of *ulcerative colitis*, in which the large intestine forms ulcers, and for *Crohn's Disease*, an autoimmune disease in which the large intestine becomes highly inflamed and ulcerated.

Like Plaquenil, described previously, sulfasalazine is prescribed in milder cases of RA. It shows some positive effects after up to two to three months in over 30 percent of people who take the tablets. There may be moderate side effects, including anemia and stomach upset, and it should not be taken by people with kidney or liver disease, asthma, or during pregnancy.

Despite its intended use as an antibacterial, there is no good evidence that this is its mode of action, and the reason for the effectiveness of sulfasalazine has yet to be determined.

Gold

If the use of antimalarials or antibacterials might strike one as an unlikely treatment for RA, then how about giving gold compounds by injection, or in capsules? Once again, the historical roots of an RA therapy go back to a time of uninformed speculation about what might be causing RA. In the late 1920s in France, Dr. Jacques Forestier started to treat his patients with RA by injecting them with gold, based on the idea that RA might be caused by tuberculosis, for which gold was one of the many attempted cures.

Over the next twenty years gold injections at rather high concentrations often proved to be quite effective against RA, but with far too many side effects, including mouth sores, skin rashes, and serious kidney problems. By the late 1940s lower doses were being prescribed, and when studies showed that these caused fewer side effects, gold was used more often. After a delay of about two to three months after beginning therapy, about 60 percent experienced a welcome reduction of pain and inflammation. In the 1980s a capsule became available, allowing easy oral administration of gold for fairly mild, slowly progressive RA.

Oral gold, as auranofin (Ridaura) has fewer side effects than injectable gold, as gold sodium thiomalate (Myochrysine), or aurothioglucose (Solganal), but is less effective. Gold is used far less now than in the past, given the increased use of methotrexate and availability of new medications (see chapter 8), and is often reserved for people who are unresponsive to other treatments.

There are a few clues as to how gold might work. The gold is taken up and concentrated in cells lining the joints, and by the macrophages, those cells that help to sustain RA in many ways—including making the inflammatory chemicals TNF-alpha and IL-1.

Penicillamine

This medication is a great example of how one has to balance the "good" news and the "bad" news about a particular therapy. In the 1960s Dr. Israeli Jaffe in New York began to use penicillamine as an RA treatment. He reasoned that this simple substance, because of its chemical structure, might be able to break up the rheumatoid factor, that protein circulating in the blood of most people with RA.

Jaffe and then many others used penicillamine (Cuprimine) with positive results. It took several months before relief became apparent, but eventually oral penicillamine proved to be as effective as gold injections, methotrexate, and sulfasalazine. That is the "good" news. The "bad" news is that penicillamine is a very toxic substance. Almost half the people who start on this drug have to stop taking it because of side effects. Those include skin eruptions, kidney problems, and blood disorders.

Now, penicillamine is reserved for people with severe, active RA who have failed to respond to the other available medications. It can be particularly useful in cases of vasculitis, a rare complication marked by inflammation of blood vessels. Research has shown that Dr. Jaffe was right—this drug does lower rheumatoid factor levels—but it's not known why or if that gives relief. Penicillamine also reduces the destructive growth of the inflamed lining in the joints, and can block other steps in the cascade of reactions in RA. Despite its effectiveness, the concern over debilitating side effects has forced penicillamine to the sidelines to be used as an agent of last resort.

Cyclosporine

For more than sixty years, chemical by-products of molds—common fungi—have been the source most of our many life-saving antibiotics, including penicillin. In 1972 a mold extract offered us another valuable drug in the form of cyclosporine. This has been used extensively since 1978, principally as a medication in connection with organ transplantion. It suppresses the immune system so that it will not reject the new organ. Based on the idea that such an inhibition of the body's defense mechanisms also might help to inhibit RA, cyclosporine has been used for RA for more than a decade in Europe.

This drug appears to have some quite specific, identifiable effects on the immune system. It is particularly effective in blocking T cells, those white blood cells that pump out lots of inflammatory chemicals, from releasing IL-2, a chemical signal that provokes inflammation in the joints. That, at least in theory, makes cyclosporine a fine candidate for slowing down RA. In 1997, the FDA approved cyclosporine for treatment of RA. However, cyclosporine as Ciclosporin and its newer formulation Neoral, a more easily absorbed solution, is seldom used by U.S. rheumatologists. It is expensive ($4,700 per year), and fairly toxic.

Despite its powerful ability to suppress certain parts of the immune system, only about one-third of those who turn to this treatment have a greater than 50 percent improvement. The side effects can be severe, especially stomach and intestinal irritation, kidney damage, and elevated blood pressure. Typically it is used in combination with methotrexate for people have severe RA and have not responded to the methotrexate alone.

Cyclophosphamide and Azathioprine

These powerful and very toxic medications are only two of the many drugs that have come out of decades of searching for anticancer compounds. Because cancerous growths contain lots of actively dividing cells, the goal has been to isolate or make chemicals that will selectively kill such cells. The ideal substance has yet to be found, but along the way some have been used with various degrees of success against cancer, and have also been applied to RA.

Chemotherapy fights cancer by trying to kill tumors. Using the same chemicals, referred to as *cytotoxic* drugs, against RA is intended to kill off rapidly dividing cells in the immune system and perhaps eliminate the cells that are driving the disease along. This kind of "shotgun" approach may slow down RA, but at a cost. Healthy cells in the body may be killed indiscriminately, causing many side effects, including serious blood disorders and infections, and may even trigger new cancerous growths.

Cyclophosphamide (Cytoxan) is more powerful and toxic than azathioprine (Imuran). It is used only when RA is severe and has not responded to other treatments, or in cases where there is severe inflammation of blood vessels (vasculitis). Aza-thioprine, while less toxic, still can trigger serious infections and blood problems. It is usually reserved for people whose RA has not responded to other DMARDs. Recently, physicians are including azathioprine in combination with other DMARDs for RA therapy.

Steroids

Perched on top of each of the body's two kidneys is a thin wedge of brown tissue, about the size of a potato chip. These small but powerful adrenal glands, in synchrony with the needs of the body, release minute amounts of dozens of different hormones, critical to the normal functioning of our cells, tissues, and organs. The inner part of the glands produce the familiar adrenaline, which increases the heart rate, blood pressure, and blood sugar levels, quickly preparing us for strenuous physical activity. The outer layer of the adrenals makes, among many other hormones, glucocorticoids.

These are more familiarly called steroid hormones, which means that they are formed from the steroid chemical choles-terol circulating in our blood. These adrenal hormones should not be confused with synthetic anabolic steroids that people take to increase the size and strength of their muscles (at risk to their health). These glucocorticoids trickling out of the adrenals into the bloodstream fine-tune our metabolism—they can speed up the breakdown of fat and proteins, raise our blood sugar, and increase sugar storage in our muscles. Our interest here is in the effects that they have on the immune system.

The principal glucocorticoid hormone is cortisol. This is an anti-inflammatory substance that the body uses to decrease the number of white blood cells and to stifle the secretion of inflammatory chemicals from tissues. Most people are more familiar with the term *cortisone*. That is the name of another adrenal hormone that the adrenal first converts into cortisol, and also is the name given to one of the several synthetic (made in the laboratory) forms of cortisol. Cortisone and other synthetics have become central to the treatment of RA, as well as other inflammatory conditions. For convenience we will use the more familiar term cortisone.

Cortisone entered the medical scene through the Herculean labors of Dr. Philip S. Hench and his colleagues at the Mayo Clinic in Rochester, Minnesota. Based on the familiar observations that some people who became pregnant or jaundiced experienced some relief from their RA, Hench guessed that there might be something produced by the body under those circumstances, possibly a hormone, whose power might be harnessed to fight the seemingly irreversible progression of RA.

By 1938, after nine years of painstaking work, they had isolated six distinct hormones from the adrenal glands of cows. An educated guess that one of those hormones might be the one they were after led them on an additional seven-year effort to extract and purify enough of it to treat someone with RA. Finally, in September 1948, a twenty-nine-year-old woman with RA was given three injections from Hench's precious supply of cortisone. Overnight, her symptoms disappeared, and she got up and walked away from the bed where she had been immobilized for four years.

As more people experienced the same miraculous transformation, the astonishing news spread around the world. In 1950, Philip Hench and his Mayo colleague Edward C. Kendall, along with Swiss biochemist Tadeus Reichstein, who had contributed to the isolation of cortisone, were awarded the Nobel Prize in Physiology or Medicine.

Unfortunately, one might even say tragically, just as in the case of many of the medications described earlier in this chapter that would follow over the years as treatments for RA, this medical "miracle" was revealed as yet another "devil's bar-

gain." As cortisone and pharmaceuticals made in the laboratory to mimic cortisone's effects were used to fight RA as well
as other conditions like asthma, serious drawbacks soon
became apparent. The unmistakable relief from pain and suffering wrought by large doses of these medications for
extended periods of time inflicts a range of serious side effects
including diabetes, dangerously high blood pressure, weight
gain, thinning of the bones (*osteoporosis*) to the point where
they fracture easily, infections, and depression. It was soon
evident that a balance had to be struck between the real benefits and the real dangers of these hormones.

Over the intervening years a debate has continued over the
use of glucocorticoids. When should they be administered,
how much, and for how long? Do they really slow down the
progression of damage in the joints? Pharmaceutical companies have created synthetic forms of these hormones—such as
the commonly prescribed prednisone, four times as potent as
cortisone, and dexamethasone, thirty times as potent. As the
debate goes on in medical journals and at conferences, in
their day-to-day practice most physicians carefully use cortisone for many people with RA. It is usually in the form of
prednisone, to calm down pain, swelling, and inflammation
in order to improve "quality of life"—certainly a valid and welcome aim of rheumatology treatment. The term "quality of
life" is a rather vague-sounding phrase. In practical terms it
may mean the difference between having to stay seated or
walking, being able once again to change a baby's diapers,
wash the dishes, or perhaps even simply comb one's hair.

Because of the potentially devastating effects of cortisone,
there are general guidelines for its use. When NSAIDs are not
able to control symptoms, and DMARDs like methotrexate are
given but have not yet taken effect, low doses of glucocorticoid
tablets can halt the symptoms in the interim. This is called
bridge therapy. Sometimes, when neither the combination of

NSAIDs and DMARDs is effective, physicians add low doses of glucocorticoids to the mix. Ideally, one uses the lowest effective dose for the shortest possible time. Sometimes severe complications of RA require much higher doses. Glucocorticoids also are injected directly into very swollen, painful joints, giving relief for several weeks without wide-ranging side effects.

Research published in 1999 offered some encouraging news. People taking only 5 milligrams of the synthetic glucocorticoid prednisolone for two years showed a sustained improvement of disease symptoms, and had no significant bone loss. Recent studies also have revealed some of the secrets of exactly why glucocorticoids have such stunning anti-inflammatory effects. In chapters 4 and 5 we discussed the role of genes in RA and the schemes under development for finding and possibly controlling those genes. When cortisone and its synthetic forms like prednisone or prednisolone come in contact with cells, that meeting turns on certain genes in the cells so that they make anti-inflammatory proteins, and it turns off other genes that are making inflammatory substances.

This kind of detailed information about how a medication works is more than just an interesting tidbit of scientific information. Knowing what happens at the level of the cell allows pharmaceutical companies to develop new forms of these hormones that can be fine-tuned to control the disease process without setting off other reactions leading to unwanted side effects.

Antibiotics

With the clarity of hindsight, it was probably unfortunate that the question of whether or not antibiotics might help to alleviate or even eliminate RA has been clouded by the controversy generated by the claims of Thomas McPherson Brown, M.D. In 1938 Dr. Brown, then at the Rockefeller Institute in New York, reported isolating peculiar bacteria, called mycoplasmas, from rheumatoid tissues. Over fifty years ago Brown, as a physician in Arlington, Virginia, began treating people with RA using the antibiotic tetracycline in its various forms, which were known to kill off mycoplasmas. He and his colleagues, notably Harold Clark, Ph.D., championed the use of antibiotics under the assumption that these bacteria were causing the RA, and so RA was best dealt with by getting rid of the bacteria.

Tales of remissions and cures abounded as Brown treated at least ten thousand people over the next four decades until his death in 1989. However, the dogged insistence on mycoplasmas as the cause of RA weakened Brown's claims. Despite years of research, there has been no clear-cut evidence that mycoplasmas or any other bacteria or virus causes RA. Of course, lack of proof does not eliminate the possibility that someday, someone might find a microbial cause. And after all, both gold and sulfasalazine, discussed earlier in this chapter, were first used against RA because they were antibacterial.

One of the reasons that Brown's claims were downplayed was because the data on his treatments, said to be successful, were not published in a respected journal in the rigorous format required by scientists. This would include precise details about such aspects as the medical histories of the patients, the dosages used, the length of treatment, and the methods used to judge results. Brown did report his results at an international meeting in Sydney, Australia, in 1985.

In addition to the criticism directed at Brown, other studies on the role that antibiotics might possibly play in RA treatment appeared sporadically over the years with few encouraging signs. However, in the early 1990s researchers in the Netherlands and in Israel reported that giving minocycline, a laboratory-synthesized form of tetracycline, gave substantial symptomatic relief. This led to more extensive trials in the Netherlands and in the United States, reported in 1994 and

1995, which concluded that minocycline did indeed reduce joint pain and swelling and had few side effects. In 1995, Michael D. Lockshin, then acting director at the National Institute of Arthritis and Musculoskeletal Diseases (NIAMS), remarked that "minocycline is another drug to add to the armamentarium of treatments for rheumatoid arthritis."

There was still widespread skepticism in the medical community, as indicated by the fact that the 1996 "Guidelines for the Management of Rheumatoid Arthritis" prepared by the ACR, does not mention antibiotics as an RA treatment.

However, an August 1999 report in the ACR journal, *Arthritis and Rheumatism*, added impetus to the growing notion that minocycline should take its place alongside the more standard therapies (discussed in this chapter). Significant aspects of this report were that the forty-six people treated were in the early stage of RA, and their progress was followed for four years. The authors concluded that "minocycline appears to be an effective therapy for early RA; further investigation into its mechanism of action is needed . . . there may be a window of opportunity early in RA, in which minocycline can produce dramatic benefit."

A careful look at the process of inflammation and damage in RA reveals one of the reasons why confusion reigned over the effect of these antibiotics. The tetracycline group, including minocycline and doxycycline, as Minocin and Doxy (among several other U.S. brand names), does not just inhibit bacterial growth, it also interferes with production of inflammatory prostaglandin chemicals and T cells in the joints. In addition, they reduce the supply of destructive enzymes that can erode cartilage and bone. Whatever beneficial effects these antibiotics have may be due to their influence on the immune system.

Further studies are needed to determine exactly how the tetracyclines affect the RA process, but despite a residue of reluctance to use these antibiotics, rheumatologists are beginning to reconsider them as a valid and useful ingredient in their combination of RA therapies. Meanwhile, a not-for-profit, all-volunteer corporation founded by "disciples" of Dr. Brown, the Road Back Foundation, at www.roadback.org, continues to boost the idea that RA is caused by mycoplasmas and related bacteria.

Drug Decisions

Beginning in the late 1980s, the more traditional "pyramid" approach to the treatment of RA was challenged by the positive results of more aggressive strategies. Typically, physicians would give someone diagnosed with RA aspirin or other NSAIDs, the "base" of the pyramid. When this therapy no longer controlled symptoms, they would switch to a DMARD—methotrexate, sulfasalazine, etc.—with the hope that this would alleviate symptoms and slow the progression of damage to the joints. If that proved ineffective, perhaps several years after the diagnosis, they would move to the "tip"—combinations of DMARDs or experimental therapies.

The idea behind the pyramid approach was that the more powerful DMARDs are more toxic, and so people should not take them until they "earned" them, that is, until their disease did not respond to NSAIDs. As careful studies revealed that bone and joint erosion can develop only after a couple of months of experiencing RA symptoms, it became apparent that earlier, more aggressive treatment was needed if there was any hope of stopping or at least slowing down the pace of the damage.

In the early 1990s the "step-down bridge" was proposed. This began with a fast-acting steroid plus methotrexate. When (and if) inflammation was reduced, the physician discontinued the steroid and methotrexate and replaced them with a milder drug, such as hydroxychloroquine. The aim was to control inflammation early before extensive joint damage could take place.

Others suggested the "sawtooth" strategy. Here, one DMARD is used early, and as it loses effect it is replaced with another DMARD. On this regime, people move up and down in a pattern like the teeth in a saw, from the heights of effectiveness to low levels of therapeutic value, and back up to more relief.

The newest approach to RA treatment is one in which combinations of DMARDs are used in the early stages of the disease. Just as in the case of cancer, early diagnosis and intervention are now considered essential to improving the long-term outcomes in people with RA. Many rheumatologists now maintain that therapy with DMARDs should begin as soon as a diagnosis of RA is made. There is a growing consensus that confronting RA in an early phase with powerful medications could make an enormous difference in avoiding disease progression and perhaps induce long-lasting remission, or at least slow down the advance of the disease.

There is an ongoing interchange of ideas within the worldwide rheumatology community about how best to translate this concept into specific treatment plans. In other words, what are the optimal combinations of drugs to use for a particular person? What signs and symptoms indicate that a specific combination might be better than another? What is the best way to diagnose RA early, and to predict which people are more likely to develop persistent and more serious damage? When is it better to "step up," that is, add DMARDs one after the other as they become ineffective, or to "step down," meaning using combinations of DMARDs right away, including steroids? Also, what is the most accurate way to monitor disease activity and assess damage? Newer, more sensitive methods of looking into joints, such as ultrasound, magnetic resonance imaging (MRI), and machines that measure bone mineral density are under investigation.

While this interchange of ideas is underway, and research reports are published and perused, the use of DMARDs in combination has become commonplace. In the United States, in early 2000 an estimated 24 percent of people being treated for RA were on combination DMARD therapy. The most common combinations were methotrexate-hydroxychloroquine, methotrexate-sulfasalazine, and methotrexate-hydroxychloroquine-sulfasalazine.

✛   ✛   ✛

The decision on the optimum treatment plan for a particular person with RA is based on many factors. It is encouraging that research continues to reveal clues that assist in that decision. One message coming out of that research is that RA responds better to early treatment. It is as though there is a window of opportunity for the most effective treatment. The earlier the treatment, the better the chance for success.

But that's not all. In contrast to only two new FDA drug approvals for RA since the late 1980s (methotrexate and cyclosporine), during 1998–1999 five brand-new, innovative medications were added to the rheumatology medicine cabinet. Two of these are less toxic, strong NSAIDs targeted at the painful signs and symptoms of RA. One is a novel, effective DMARD and the other two represent an entirely new class of medications designed to block essential steps leading to inflammation and joint damage. Let's look at what these newcomers add to our progress toward conquering RA.

CHAPTER 8

The New Medicines

According to the authors of a 1937 text on the latest "advances" in the treatment of the various forms of arthritis, "Rheumatologists as a class are optimistic; the chronic and progressive character of rheumatism makes it imperative that they should be so, otherwise they would often feel inclined to give up treatment in despair." The rheumatologists of the time, and especially the people they were trying to help, had little more than optimism on their side. However, as the numbers and kinds of medications for treating RA have increased over the decades, cautious optimism is realistic.

As we saw in chapter 7, new medications may arrive on the scene with great promise, only to have that promise tempered with the realization that they are not useful for everyone. Too often, the great relief that they give is accompanied by serious side effects that severely limit their use. Drugs that bring relief in the beginning become ineffective over time. However, despite the fact that "the cure" for RA has not yet appeared, the opportunities for people with RA at the beginning of the twenty-first century are a world apart from the lack of any real treatments in 1937. For many people, timely and careful use of the medications, described in the chapter 7, has eased their pain, slowed the progress of their disease, and improved the quality of their lives in a way that would have seemed miraculous in earlier years.

During 1998–1999, there were more reasons for optimism in the form of FDA approval of five new medications and a unique therapeutic device. Leflunomide (Arava), arrived in 1998 as a new, useful DMARD. Nineteen ninety-nine marked the arrival of two novel NSAIDs, celecoxib (Celebrex) and rofecoxib (Vioxx), the second of which was approved for use in osteoarthritis, but was expected to be applied to RA at some later date. These are unique NSAIDs in that they provide the pain relief similar to other NSAIDs , such as ibuprofen, but with a lower incidence of gastrointestinal problems. Also in 1999, the Prosorba column, a blood-filtering device, became available to treat people in the most severe stages of RA.

One of the most imposing challenges to the optimism of rheumatologists has been the management of "refractory" RA, which means disease that does not respond adequately to any treatment. People in this situation endure pain and disability that profoundly compromise their quality of life. Two new and unique medications, which employ novel strategies for interfering directly with crucial pathways in the inner workings of the RA disease process, have raised new hopes that the burden borne by many people with refractory RA will be significantly reduced.

Etanercept (Enbrel) and infliximab (Remicade), approved in late 1998 and 1999, respectively, are both aimed at blocking the malicious effects of TNF-alpha. This chemical, one of the most important cytokines (small proteins used by cells to communicate with each other) in RA, unleashes a whole cascade of inflammatory reactions that enhances and perpetuates joint damage. With these medications, we have entered a new age of relatively safe, effective *biologics* in RA treatment. Biologics are medications based on compounds that are made

by living cells, rather than medications synthesized chemically, as is done to prepare conventional pharmaceuticals like
aspirin or methotrexate.

The positive (yet cautious, as we shall see) responses by
rheumatologists to the appearance of these new medications
certainly were shared by the manufacturers of these novel
products. Total sales of RA therapies in 1999 worldwide was
almost $1.5 billion. With the advent of the new NSAIDs, the
adoption of unique biologics, and the promise of others to
follow (see chapter 9), estimates of $6.6 billion by 2009, with
$4.5 billion of that in biologics sales alone, seem realistic.

Impressive sales by pharmaceutical companies, of course,
translate at the consumers' end to impressive costs. Indeed,
legitimate concern over the high cost of some of these new
medications is a particularly poignant problem that factors
into a long list of considerations surrounding the selection of
medication(s) to use in any particular case. These recent
arrivals, hailed as significant new treatment options, bring
with them different promises and precautions. The publicity
surrounding their approval by the FDA for use against RA has
been a mixture of hype and hope. Let's look at the relevant
facts about each one of them. In keeping with the public
interest that each has generated, and in tune with the times,
each has its own Web site.

COX FIGHTING

We pointed out in chapter 7 that the traditional NSAIDs, such
as ibuprofen or aspirin, give us some relief from inflammation and pain by interfering with the activity of a common
enzyme, abbreviated as COX. This enzyme is responsible for
making chemicals called prostaglandins, some of which are
beneficial in our tissues, while others are harmful. In RA the

inflamed joints make lots of the prostaglandins that contribute to the pain and inflammation.

Researchers discovered that there are two distinct forms of the COX enzyme, COX-1 and COX-2 (see www.cox2.org). Finding that the COX-2 form makes the kinds of prostaglandins that are very active in RA, they set about to find a substance that could block only COX-2. That's because the COX-1 type of enzyme is always active in our tissues, making prostaglandins that help to maintain the healthy functioning of our kidneys, lungs, and gastrointestinal tract. The typical NSAIDs, to varying degrees, slow down both types of COX. This means that while NSAIDs are providing welcome relief, they also reduce the amount of helpful prostaglandins, particularly in the stomach. This sometimes leads to irritation or even ulceration and bleeding in the stomach lining. A 1997 study listed 16,500 NSAID- related deaths among the 100,000 NSAID-related hospital admissions. Because so many people with RA take these medications, NSAID users endure an estimated 20,000 hospitalizations and 2,600 deaths per year from stomach complications.

The toll that NSAIDs take on the stomach is due to the fact that they cut down on the amount of protective prostaglandins, which normally inhibit acid secretion and protect the stomach lining with a layer of thick mucus. NSAIDs increase the acid secretion and interfere with mucus production.

Not everyone taking NSAIDs runs the same risks. There are variables to consider such as the specific drug, the dose, the duration of exposure to the medication, and, as usual, the great variety of individual characteristics of the people who take the drug, including age (over sixty increases risk) and tendency to develop stomach ulcers.

Taking NSAIDs is a trade-off between benefits and possible harm. Taking this calculated risk is by no means unusual. Three hundred million people worldwide are estimated as using NSAIDs, making it the most frequently prescribed class of medication. Of course, some NSAIDs, like ibuprofen and aspirin, are available over the counter. In the United States, 1.2 percent of the population takes NSAIDs daily, consuming over 40 billion aspirins and 70 million NSAID prescriptions yearly. In addition to being used routinely for RA, they are a mainstay of treatment for osteoarthritis and a variety of other conditions such as musculoskeletal injuries, gout, and everyday aches and pains.

Is it any wonder that the launching of Celebrex, approved by the FDA on December 31, 1998, as the first-ever specific COX-2 inhibitor, generated enormous excitement? In the first fifteen weeks, more prescriptions were written for Celebrex than for any other new drug in the history of the pharmaceutical industry—including even Viagra, the famed anti-impotence drug, which ran a close second. Over the next two years, more than 21 million Celebrex prescriptions would be filled.

Marketed by Pharmacia Corporation's Searle, Skokie, Illinois (www.pharmacia.com), and Pfizer, Inc., New York, New York (www.pfizer.com), Celebrex (www.celebrex.com), despite its immediate popularity, nevertheless met with some early challenges over its claims of safety versus traditional NSAIDs. There had been a number of studies comparing its relative safety before the FDA gave its final approval, but questions were raised about the possible long-term effects of Celebrex.

However, by mid-September 2000, the results were compiled and publicized on studies with Celebrex involving 8059 subjects over a six-month period. The dose used was higher than that recommended for RA (which, for the latter, is 200 mg twice daily), and the effects were compared other NSAIDs. In those tested (omitting those who were taking aspirin) the relative risks for ulcers and ulcer complications were 1.4 percent for Celebrex and 2.91 percent for the NSAIDs.

When these and other studies looked at the relative effec-

tiveness of Celebrex versus other NSAIDs, including diclo-
fenac, naproxen sodium (Naprosyn), and ibuprofen, in relieving the pain and inflammation of RA, Celebrex was about
equal to the other drugs tested. However, with Celebrex there
was an overall significantly lower incidence of undesirable
side effects such as abdominal pain and nausea.

These data indicate that Celebrex may be the least dangerous NSAID. As the same data show, the real possibility still
exists for uncomfortable and sometimes serious complications. As usual for any drug, there is a list of cautions to be
observed. For example, Celebrex should be used with caution
in people with kidney disease or high blood pressure.

As we have pointed out several times, decisions as to which
NSAID to prescribe for a person with RA encompass many different considerations, such as the person's age and general
health, among others. There is also the issue of cost. In the
United States, about 70 percent of people with RA have health
insurance through managed care organizations. These health
plans differ in regard to who covers the cost of various medical
therapies. The cost of taking Celebrex averages about $2.50 per
day, as compared to ibuprofen, which costs about 20 cents a
day. At an annual cost of about $900, people without health
insurance and those whose insurance does not cover their
entire expenses may have a real problem.

Health maintenance organizations (HMOs) claim to share
in their version of the cost dilemma. For example, a major
HMO in the northeastern United States calculated that if half
their clients on traditional NSAIDs were to switch to Celebrex,
the increased cost could reach $18.6 million per year. However,
the drugs makers argue that HMOs will actually save money by
cutting down on the hospitalizations resulting from NSAID-
related ulcers and reduce the need for medications used to
counter NSAID side effects.

Celebrex is the least expensive of the new RA medications

described in this chapter. Even so, using Celebrex may be a financial burden. There is a toll-free number available ([800] 542-2526) to ask for an application for financial assistance to purchase Celebrex (your doctor's call is required).

There are other COX-2 inhibitors in the marketplace. Rofecoxib (Vioxx), (www.vioxx.com), manufactured by Merck and Co., Whitehouse Station, New Jersey (www.merck.com), was given FDA approval in May 1999 for use in acute pain and osteoarthritis. Meloxicam (Mobic), from Boehringer Ingelheim Pharmaceuticals, Ingelheim, Germany (www.boehringer-ingelheim.com), and Abbott Laboratories, Abbott Park, Illinois (www.abbott.com), received FDA approval in April 2000 as a treatment for osteoarthritis. Developed in the early 1990s, Mobic was the first specific COX-2 inhibitor, and has been available since then in in Europe. In December 2000, Canada approved meloxicam, as Mobicox, for use in RA as well as osteoarthritis. Both Vioxx and Mobic have been shown to be safer than conventional NSAIDs.

The story of COX-2 has not been confined to its important role in inflammation. Research on the wider role of COX-2 has led to some remarkable discoveries and possibilities. For over twenty years there has been an accumulation of studies showing that anti-inflammatory substances might have an anti-cancer effect. There were no satisfactory theories as to why this might happen until June 2000, when the *New England Journal of Medicine* reported the effects of Celebrex on seventy-seven volunteers with a serious, inherited, precancerous disorder. They had a condition that causes hundreds of polyps, small masses of tissue, to grow inside their large intestines, virtually guaranteeing that if the polyps are not removed, colon cancer will develop. After six months of treatment with Celebrex, there was significant decrease in the number of these polyps.

Many questions still need to be answered on the effects of COX-2 in people at high risk for cancer. Meanwhile, as those studies continue, other research is looking at the potential role of COX-2 inhibition in Alzheimer's disease and stroke. The future of the current crop of COX-2 inhibitors and their successors looks promising indeed.

Beyond pharmaceuticals, there may be a more "natural" form of inflammation control. Studies have suggested that an ingredient in fish oils—the Omega-3 fatty acids—can help reduce inflammation in the joints. A possible explanation may be that these substances, found in cod liver and other fish oils, and in highest concentrations in salmon, mackerel, and other cold-water varieties, become incorporated into cartilage cells within the joints. There, they reduce the activity of COX-2 enzymes, and thereby decrease pain and inflammation.

Whatever associations there might be between one's diet and the symptoms of RA, in the final analysis any connection comes down once again to the chemical reactions that go on in our cells and tissues. There are many still unanswered questions about these potential links, or for that matter about other substances reputed to be effective against RA. A guide to those issues is found in *The Arthritis Foundation Guide to Alternative Therapies*, available by calling (800) 207-8633 or at www.arthritis.org.

A New DMARD

September 1, 1998, marked the first FDA approval of a new RA medication in over ten years. Leflunomide (Arava; www.arava. com), from Aventis Pharmaceuticals, Inc., Parsippany, New Jersey (www.aventispharma-us.com), became a welcome member of the DMARDs, those "disease-modifying antirheumatic drugs" that we described in chapter seven. Leflunomide, approved for use in active RA in adults (even for those who may not have failed prior DMARD therapies) works differently from the other DMARDs, such as methotrexate or sulfasalazine.

Although leflunomide's mode of action is not yet completely understood (which we have seen is true for most RA medications), it is known to reduce the number of T cells, those specialized white blood cells that contribute to the damaging effects and painful symptoms of RA. It does this by inhibiting the activity of a particular enzyme used in a pathway leading to active T cell formation. It also appears to slow down the activity of enzymes that break down cartilage and bone.

Among the other DMARDs, methotrexate is generally regarded as somwhat more effective than sulfasalazine. Leflunomide compares favorably with both of these medications. Like them, leflunomide can slow down the rate of damage to affected joints. In October 2000, the report of a twenty-four-week study of 263 volunteers who were not responding to methotrexate showed that 46 percent of those who were given leflunomide along with methotrexate experienced significant relief.

Interestingly, in a yearlong study comparing leflunomide with methotrexate—the latter being the standard against which other DMARDs are generally judged—among 482 people with RA, those who took leflunomide experienced significantly more improvement in an important category. Evaluations of the relative improvement in the subject's "quality of life," such as her capacity to conduct daily activities—e.g., walking, eating, dressing, and washing—and her sense of "well-being" indicated that leflunomide appeared to be superior to methotrexate.

As anyone with RA knows, any chance for improvement in these kinds of simple activities, often taken for granted by people who do not have to endure the pain and stiffness of RA, merits serious consideration. And as usual, there are other considerations to keep in mind. Leflunomide doesn't work for everyone. About 40 to 65 percent of the people who take this medication show improvement. There may be side effects including abdominal pain, diarrhea, loss of appetite, and (reversible) hair loss. Liver function has to be monitored on a regular basis, and leflunomide must not be taken during pregnancy. Males who are considering fathering a child are advised to avoid it as well.

Leflunomide therapy begins usually with one 100 milligram tablet for three days, and then a 20 millgram tablet once a day. This simple regimen bears a monthly cost of about $245, amounting to an annual total of around $2,940 (financial assistance applications are available at [800] 552-3656). Because of the hefty expense, leflunomide may not soon replace methotrexate as the DMARD of choice, but certainly is a potentially effective addition for people who do not respond to methotrexate alone. Studies contiue that will lead to a clearer understanding of how this unique DMARD can play a role in the emerging emphasis on early aggressive treatment of RA, including how it might be best combined with other medications for optimum effect.

A Novel Approach

Diseases desperate grown
By desperate appliance are reliev'd
Or not at all.

These few lines from Shakespeare's *Hamlet* might seem to apply to the first nondrug therapy for RA to be approved by the FDA. On March 16, 1999, that agency sanctioned the use of the Prosorba column, a blood-filtering device. This method is recommended only for those with moderate to severe RA who have not experienced significant relief from DMARDs. But while many of those people who fit that description might sometimes consider themselves desperate, the Prosorba device is really quite simple.

According to the manufacturer of the Prosorba column (www.prosorba.com), Cypress Bioscience, San Diego, California (www.cypressbio.com), between two and five hundred thousand people with RA in the United States alone could benefit from this treatment. The technique for treatment with the column is quite a departure from daily doses of medication. Each week for twelve weeks, one reports to a clinic or a doctor's office, where, in a two-hour procedure, one's blood flows through tubing attached to an arm vein into an apheresis machine—a cell separator. This separates the liquid part of the blood (the plasma) from the blood cells. The plasma then passes through the Prosorba column, about the size and shape of a soup can, out through another tube, where it is reunited with the blood cells and returned to you through a vein in the other arm.

In other words, your blood cells wait while the blood plasma is "filtered," and then the plasma and cells are returned to you. The procedure filters about four to eight cups of plasma over the two-hour period. Actually, the term "filter" is not an accurate reflection of what goes on in the column. In fact, the column is yet another example of an RA treatment that can be effective, but for reasons that are not entirely clear.

The Prosorba column had been in FDA-approved use for ten years for idiopathic thrombocytic purpurea (ITP; www.itppeople.com), an autoimmune blood disorder that affects one hundred thousand people in the United States. In this disease the body's immune system attacks and destroys the blood platelets, tiny cell fragments that allow the blood to clot normally. Among other problems, this can cause serious bleeding. Some people with this disorder are helped by being treated with the Prosorba column, and over the years, some individuals under treatment for ITP also experienced some relief from their RA symptoms.

There are various techniques for separating someone's blood into its components, treating the components, and returning the altered blood. Some of these methods have been tried over the years for RA as well as other autoimmune disorders such as lupus. The logic behind these trials is that notion that there are troublesome components in blood, such as the protein rheumatoid factor or clumps of combined antigens and antibodies called "immune complexes," that might be removed from the blood by apheresis.

The original reasoning behind the beneficial effects of the Prosorba column was based on the properties of its absorbent material. The column is a plastic cylinder packed with a grainy silica filling, which is coated with protein A, a protein derived from a special variety of *Staphylococcus* bacteria. This protein A can bind to antibodies and antigen-antibody complexes. It seemed that this would be an effective way to grab those potentially inflammatory substances in the blood plasma as it flowed through the column. As it turns out, relatively minute amounts of these substances are removed by the column. Something else must be happening, and scientific analyses are underway to understand further how Prosorba actually works.

If you were one of the sixteen out of forty-eight people with RA who showed a 20 percent or greater improvement in their signs and symptoms after they participated in the 1998 tests of the Prosorba column, the intimate details of what protein A was doing to your blood might not seem very important. It might fade in significance, particularly when the improvement after the Prosorba treatments last an average of thirty-seven weeks and up to seventy-five weeks in some cases.

All of the volunteers for these trials had endured RA for an average of fifteen years, and had tried more than five different DMARDs. As a matter of fact, because the Prosorba treatment was so effective, the trials were cut short so that the treatment could be made available earlier to those who might be helped by it. This was the first time that a trial for an RA treatment had been stopped early because the benefits were so obvious.

Another encouraging aspect of this treatment is that in the 1998 study, 78 percent of the people who had responded positively to the twelve-week course of Prosorba treatment responded again when they went through another treatment series. As with any RA treatment, there are side effects that can occur through the use of the Prosorba column. They are usually temporary and manageable, and include chills and fever. People undergoing treatment often experience fatigue and an increase in joint pain and swelling for a day or two. All of the side effects at this point appear to be reversible and are related to the apheresis procedure, and not to the use of the column itself.

Again, there is the cost consideration. A series of twelve monthly treatments averages a total of about $20,000. Fortunately, in June, 2000 the U.S. Health Care Financing Administration (HFCA; www.hfca.gov), decided to expand Medicare coverage to include Prosorba column therapy. Questions about insurance coverage for Prosorba can be directed to (800) 255-7277.

The fact that we do not know the details of how the Prosorba column can sometimes bring welcome relief is not a trivial consideration. When the puzzle is solved it may lead to a more efficient way to attack RA that can be applied to more people and at a much earlier stage of the disease. The fact that the results of this therapy can include the remarkable stories of the two young women featured on the Prosorba Web site, whose lives were transformed by treatment, and also the majority of the others treated for whom the results were modest at best, underscores again the frustrating, complex nature of RA.

The Prosorba column therapy is not for everyone. As research continues on how to expand its use beyond the most seriously afflicted, it does at least offer the possibility of some relief from pain and disability.

FIGHTING THE FACTOR

The various therapies for RA, as we have seen, while often effective for some, have not been based on specific, detailed knowledge of how that therapy—NSAIDs, DMARDs, and so on—can interfere with a particular, crucial step in the process of inflammation. In other words, if the cells and chemical pathways causing the stiffness, pain, and eventually the joint damage of RA are the target of our therapies, we are using a shotgun to hit the target instead of a rifle. The shotgun pellets may hit the target, but can damage lots of other objects in the area—so we get unwanted side effects. If we could use a rifle and take dead aim at the target, we could hit it and nothing else.

The era of "rifle" therapy is much closer with two new "biologic" medications, referred to in the beginning of this chapter as the type of medications based on chemicals made by living cells. Not only are these biologics "natural" rather than synthetic chemicals, they represent a new strategy. Recall that the "words" cells use (in our case, immune system cells) to communicate with each other is in the form of chemicals—the cytokines. These are small protein molecules that cells make and release into their immediate environment. The cytokines influence other cells in the area when the special receptors on the outer membranes of those cells detect their presence. This meeting of cytokines and receptors sets off a series of reactions that, in the case of RA, can lead to inflammation, swelling, pain, and damage. The strategy of the new biologics is to block those cytokines.

We have often mentioned one of the cytokines central to RA—tumor necrosis factor-alpha, usually shortened to TNF-alpha. Its name comes from the fact that this cytokine can kill tumor cells under certain conditions; in other words, make them undergo "necrosis," meaning death. TNF-alpha is a vital member of the group of at least twenty-four different cytokines that drive the destructive reactions in RA.

Remember, these cytokines play an important role in maintaining normal health. They are produced in response to infection or injury and stimulate our immune systems to fight back. Unfortunately, in RA, the natural control mechanisms that normally turn off the immune response after it has done its job are unable to do so. We do not yet know all the details of why this happens, but we know, for example, that uncontrolled TNF-alpha is a serious troublemaker. It can transform cells in the synovium, the delicate membrane lining the joints, into a growing, invading mass of tissue—the pannus—that eats away at the cartilage and bone. It also attracts more inflammatory cells to the area, aids in the formation of additional small blood vessels, and helps make enzymes that can break down cartilage and bone.

The major source of TNF-alpha are the macrophages—plentiful, active cells that move around in the joint tissues. The macrophages' normal assignment is to pick up material in the tissues that the body recognizes as foreign and dangerous to it, like bacteria or perhaps pieces of injured cells. The macrophages, carrying these foreign fragments—called antigens—come in contact with special kinds of white blood cells, the T cells. This meeting stimulates the T cells to make cytokines that attract other T cells and macrophages to the site. Soon there is an abundant supply of TNF-alpha coming from the macrophages, which can transform joint cells to divide and destroy. In addition, TNF-alpha induces other cells in the area to make inflammatory cytokines, like inter-leukin-1 (IL-1) and interleukin-6 (IL-6).

Under ordinary conditions, if we develop a minor bacterial infection in a hand, for example, we may experience some local redness, swelling, and pain that may persist for a few days, and then disappear. The macrophages, T cells, and the cytokines have done their work, and then they slow down until the next invasion. We do not know the exact trigger(s) that begin this inflammatory process in RA, but we do know that our challenge is to slow down its abnormal, destructive continuation.

That is why a therapy aimed directly at reducing the amount and activity of TNF-alpha makes sense. Fortunately, we have been able to gain some understanding of the TNF-alpha control system that the immune system normally uses. When molecules of TNF-alpha are released by cells like macrophages, the soluble molecules can attach to special protein receptors on the surface of cells in the joint, such as cells in the synovial membrane, or cells that line the tiny blood vessels in the area. Once attached to the receptors on these cells, the TNF-alpha induces the cells (by turning on some of their genes) to keep the inflammation going. In the fluid surrounding these cells there is a variable amount of those protein TNF-alpha receptors that are free-floating. These are part of the natural control system, because they can grab onto TNF-alpha and thereby not allow it to bind to receptors on cells, which causes the inflammation. This allows some "fine-tuning" of the effects of TNF-alpha. However, in the joints of someone with RA, even though there are increased amounts of these dissolved receptors grabbing TNF-alpha and keeping it from making trouble, they are unable to stop it from prodding the immune system down the path of RA.

Our knowledge is expanding about the details of the complicated system of interacting cells and cytokines, which is so crucial to our health but is so damaging to it when the natural controls no longer function. How can we, as the saying goes, stick a "monkey wrench" into the works, and stop RA from progressing? Before we explain how we now have made a giant leap toward doing just that—a word of caution. Once again, RA shows its many faces—there is a wide variety of levels of TNF-alpha and other inflammatory cytokines in the joint tissues of people with RA—which may explain why the following new treatments work so well in many people with RA, but not in all.

CHALLENGING TNF-ALPHA

A new era in the fight against RA began on November 2, 1998. The FDA approved a unique drug, etanercept (Enbrel), for use in moderate to severe RA, when other treatments have not been effective. Enbrel (www.enbrel.com), from Immunex Corporation, Seattle, Washington, and Wyeth-Ayerst, Philadelphia, Pennsylvania, both divisions of American Home Products Corporation, Madison, New Jersey (www.ahp.com), became the first specific anticytokine therapy ever sanctioned for use in RA. Enbrel's cytokine target is TNF-alpha, and it aims at that target by mimicking the natural TNF-alpha receptors normally found in the body.

In other words, it is a biologic therapy, using compounds that are made by living cells rather than those that are synthesized in the laboratory. Using human cells, scientists at Immunex Corporation managed to remove and purify a batch of the gene responsible for making the natural TNF-alpha receptor proteins. They then attached those genes to other genes whose job it is to make a piece of a human antibody. When they took the gene combination that they had fastened together and put it into a batch of living, dividing animal cells, the genes entered the cells and began to do what genes are sup-

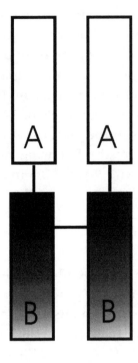

Fig. 12. A model of the novel medication Enbrel. (A) represents the part of the molecule that is a human TNF-alpha receptor. (B) represents a human antibody molecule. The fusion of (A) and (B) is etanercept, known by its brand name Enbrel. It can stop the inflammatory activity of the cytokine TNF-alpha by binding to it.

posed to do—make proteins. Those proteins are separated out from the animal cell culture and purified. The proteins that the genes make is Enbrel—a novel hybrid of human antibody–human TNF-alpha receptor (Fig. 12).

Enbrel usually is administered by self-injection twice weekly, just under the skin. When Enbrel, carried by the blood, arrives at the joints where TNF-alpha is acting up, it grabs tightly onto the TNF-alpha. This prevents the TNF-alpha from attaching to receptors on cells in the joint and starting a cascade of inflammatory reactions.

This kind of molecular manipulation of genes and cells is called *genetic engineering*. The tools of genetic engineering— gene identification and isolation; gene insertion into bacteria, plants, or animals; harvesting of the gene protein products— are now central to the modern life sciences. Stories (and controversies) over genetically modified foods or animals are now common topics in the news. Ingenious genetic manipulations are now being used for making new medications—and Enbrel is just the first in what will be a growing list of genetically engineered therapies for RA.

Trials of Enbrel leading to its FDA approval were impressive. In one trial, people who had endured RA for an average of twelve years, and had stopped responding to an average of three DMARDs, often responded favorably to Enbrel within the first two weeks. After six months, 59 percent had a greater than 20 percent improvement, 40 percent had a greater than 50 percent improvement, and 15 percent experienced relief of greater than 70 percent.

In fact, when additional results continued to underline the benefits of Enbrel, including X-ray data that showed Enbrel can slow down the progress of joint deterioration, the FDA extended its approval of Enbrel to people with moderate to severely active RA—but not limited to those who had failed DMARD therapy. In other words, physicians, after considering all the circumstances and options, can now prescribe Enbrel in the early stages of the disease, without first trying, for example, the familiar DMARD methotrexate, although Enbrel can be used in combination with methotrexate.

The FDA went a step further on August 6, 1999, when it endorsed Enbrel for use in moderately to severely active polyarticular juvenile rheumatoid arthritis (JRA), in children who have had an inadequate response to one or more DMARDs. This disease, affecting approximately seventy thousand children in the United States, strikes children before the age of sixteen. It can cause painful joint swelling, deformity, stunted growth, and increased mortality. Enbrel brought significant relief to fifty-one of sixty-nine children tested in 1998, prior to the approval. Daniel Lovell, a pediatric rheumatologist at Children's Hospital Medical Center of Cincinnati (www.cincinnatichildrens.org) and leader of this clinical study, feels that "the approval of Enbrel for JRA opens a new era of hope for these children, teen-agers, and their familes."

One of the important questions always asked about an RA medication is whether or not people taking it will continue to respond favorably to it over an extended period of time. People can become *refractory* to a medication, that is, even though they continue to take it, the drug becomes less effective. In October 2000, a welcome report on a large-scale study of people with active RA revealed that those who responded to Enbrel had experienced reduction of joint pain and swelling for as long as four years of treatment. After thirty months of treatment, among the subjects who started out with an average of thirty tender and twenty-five swollen joints, no tender joints were seen in 24 percent and no swollen joints were seen in 21 percent.

The fact that Enbrel has to be injected under the skin can be a problem for some people. Also, it is common to experience some itchy, red swelling at the injection site. Enbrel should not be used for people who have an active infection or are prone to infection. These concerns are seldom serious, and the side effects of Enbrel compared to other RA treatments are minimal. However, at about $1,190 per month, the annual bill of $14,280 is a serious consideration. The Enbrel Web site directs viewers to a reimbursement support line at (800) 282-7704, where one can talk to an insurance specialist.

Another fascinating possibility for using the genes that make Enbrel was reported by Haim Burstein of Targeted Genetics Corporation, Seattle, Washington (www.targen.com), at the 2000 meeting of the American Society of Gene Therapy. He and colleagues from the National Institutes of Health injected harmless viruses containing Enbrel genes into the joints of arthritic rats. There was a dramatic reduction in joint swelling, and injection into a joint in one limb decreased swelling in the opposite limb joint as well. It appears that the genes entered the joints and made a supply of therapeutic anti-TNF-alpha molecules. With further development of this approach we may see the day when humans with RA are given genes to produce specific anti-RA molecules where they are needed most.

ANOTHER TNF-ALPHA CHALLENGER

Enbrel is not the only way to block some of the destructive effects of that infamous cytokine TNF-alpha. In November 1999, one year after Enbrel appeared on the scene, another option was made available by the FDA in the form of infliximab (Remicade; www.remicade.com). Its designers used a very different strategy to make an antibody that could grab onto TNF-alpha and inactivate it. Remicade is marketed in the United States by Centocor, Inc., Malvern, Pennsylvania, and Ortho-McNeil Pharmaceuticals, Inc., Raritan, New Jersey, both affiliates of Johnson and Johnson, Brunswick, New Jersey (www.johnsonjohnson.com).

After the researchers injected mice with human TNF-alpha, the mice made antibodies toward it. Removing just the portion of the antibody molecule that physically binds to the TNF-alpha, they fused it to a piece of a human antibody molecule (Fig. 13). This meant that they had created antibody molecules that were mouse-human hybrids. Their reasoning was that the mouse portion would bind to TNF-alpha, while having about 75 percent of the hybrid from a human source would reduce the chances of the human recipient with RA recognizing the mouse portion and reject the mouse-human molecules.

The kinds of antibodies that the mice make against human TNF-alpha are called *monoclonal antibodies* (*Mabs*). The Nobel Prize–winning technique of getting mice to make specific antibodies against injected molecules goes back to 1975. Since that time the use of such antibodies has spread to almost every

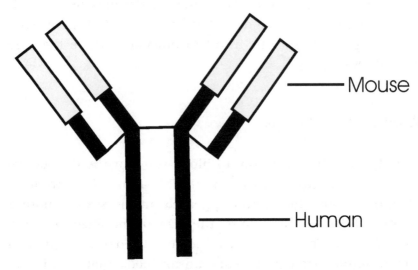

Fig. 13. A model of the novel medication Remicade. The "mouse" portion of the molecule is a TNF-alpha receptor made in mice. The "human" portion is a human antibody. The fusion of these two is infliximab, known by its brand name, Remicade. It can stop the inflammatory activity of the cytokine TNF-alpha by binding to it.

branch of biomedical research, mainly for detection and diagnosis. However, by the mid-1990s refinements in the technique led to a major expansion in research on the use of Mabs for therapy. By 2000, Mabs were under development for possible therapy against a dozen diseases including AIDS/HIV, diabetes, and especially cancer. In fact, there were over one hundred clinical trials for Mabs directed at cancer alone. With Remicade, RA joined the ranks of the human diseases targeted by these precisely aimed antibody "rifles."

The FDA approval of Remicade followed favorable results of the large-scale ATTRACT trial (Anti-TNF Trial in Rheumatoid Arthritis with Concomitant Therapy). ATTRACT studied 428 people with RA from thirty-four clinics in the United States, Canada, and Europe. The volunteers had lived with RA for an average of eight years. Their disease was actively progressing despite methotrexate therapy. The basic objective of ATTRACT was to investigate the long-term benefits of Remicade in combination with methotrexate.

At the end of fifty-four weeks, 52 percent of the subjects treated with methotrexate and Remicade had at least a 20 percent improvement, 33 percent improved 50 percent, and 18 percent showed as much as 70 percent relief—much better than those who stayed on methotrexate alone. Notably, Remicade brought noticeable relief as early as one week after initial administration. Significantly, X-ray analysis showed no progression of joint damage in 46 percent of those using Remicade—a very encouraging sign indeed. In January 2001, the FDA approved the use of Remicade in combination with methotrexate, for inhibiting the progression of structural damage in people with moderate to severely active RA who have had an inadequate response to methotrexate.

Unlike Enbrel, the other specific TNF-alpha blocker, which is given by injections under the skin, Remicade must be administered intravenously, under careful supervision. The initial dose is followed by another two and six weeks later, and then one every eight weeks thereafter. Anyone with an active infection or prone to infections cannot be given Remicade, and side effects are common, including headache, nausea, and upper respiratory tract infections. At an annual price of $7,000–$11,000 for Remicade, cost again becomes a factor. Because it is given intravenously, it meets the criteria for Medicare reimbursement. There is information about a financial assistance program at (800) 964-8345.

Rheumatologists are regarding these new and intriguing TNF-alpha blockers with cautious optimism. As more experience is gained with their use, and as other forms of cytokine antagonists become available, this novel approach will more than likely become an integral part of treatment programs aimed at gaining control over RA.

✪   ✪   ✪

So far, we have reviewed the spectrum of standard as well as new and innovative therapies for RA. Now let's take a look at what the near future may have in store, as researchers continue to refine the tools we already have, and invent new ones, to help humanity to better control and eventually conquer RA.

CHAPTER 9

Clinical Trials

t's a long, winding, and costly road from the concept of a new drug to treat a disease to the reality of having that medication available for use. Because of the rigorous safety precautions surrounding new drug approvals, and the complexities of translating an idea into a safe, effective substance, pharmaceutical companies spend approximately $400–$900 million to usher a single drug from the laboratory to the medicine cabinet. It may take ten to twelve years or more to complete that process of moving an experimental drug from "bench to bottle." Only five out of five thousand substances make it as far as clinical tests on humans. Of those five, only one eventually will be approved for sale.

This demanding and expensive process of research and development of new drugs is known in the pharmaceutical industry as the "pipeline." Lots of time, money and materials enter one end of the pipe, and eventually a few finished products trickle out the other end. In 2000, the pharmaceutical industry spent about $21 billion in research and development. However, even though companies typically invest about 15 percent of their revenues in research and development, if they manage to create a useful and widely prescribed product it may offer a quick return on their investment and generate sizeable profits. In fact, the prices of many modern drugs, including those made for RA, created by the highly sophisticated molecular techniques now available, are so high that they are out of the reach of patients without medical insurance or some form of financial assistance.

This growing gap between the haves and the have-nots extends beyond the question of who in the United States has access to the newer medications now on the market and those near the business end of the pipeline. An even wider gap exists between the developed and the developing countries. After all, the 1 percent of the population that has RA extends across the world's population of over 6 billion people, more than 1 billion of whom live in absolute poverty. These are important dilemmas, beyond the scope of this book, which will continue to test our resources, our ingenuity, and our commitment to the welfare of global humanity.

Our interest here is in looking at RA drug development and clinical testing. What medications are in the pipeline for future RA treatment, what are the steps required to add them to the medicine cabinet, including testing on humans, and how can we keep track of their progress as they move through the "pipe"?

THE FIRST STEPS

The people directing pharmaceutical research are professional scientists, usually with M.D. and/or Ph.D. degrees, who work at universities, research centers, or pharmaceutical companies. They typically work in collaboration with other scientists at the same or other institutions. Their work may be funded by governmental agencies, such as the National Institutes of Health (NIH), or by the companies that employ them.

In any case, the wide array of freely available basic research results published in hundreds of science journals and presented at science conferences is the basis for much of their initial work. Basic research is the kind of study that is not directed toward a specific treatment. It asks fundamental questions, for example, about the way in which the molecules of living systems interact, such as role of cytokines like TNF-alpha in the inflamed joint, or about which genes may be turned on before and during the onset of RA.

The ongoing accumulation and publication of this necessary, basic information about how living systems work—from the level of the whole body, down through the organ systems, the tissues, cells, genes, and finally the molecules—is a treasure chest of knowledge for scientists and a key to the potential of modern medical science. Armed with a still incomplete but always increasing knowledge of the mechanisms of diseases such as RA, the next step is to fashion a way to intervene in the disease process.

One approach, "targeted synthesis," focuses on a particular step in disease progression. Even though the target (such as an inflammatory cytokine made by white blood cells) may be known, it still may be necessary to screen hundreds of compounds before finding one that is promising. There are other approaches as well that are not as specific, such as "random screening" of thousands of chemical agents, only one or a few of which may be of some use. Sometimes a part of a compound is used as a base, and molecular segments of other agents are added to enhance its activity. In a more high-tech synthesis of "designer" drugs, researchers manipulate chemical structures by computer modeling so that the resulting molecules can fit the three-dimensional shape of a target molecule, such as a protein, and activate or deactivate it.

After these preliminaries, the next step is "discovery testing." The questions to be answered here include: Does the compound work in animals? Is it long- or short-acting? In other words, how long does it have its desired effects? They should be long enough so that the medication can be administered in one or a few doses per day, but not so long that if the person were to experience an adverse reaction, the risk and discomfort would be extended.

Ideally, the compound should have good "specificity," that is, it affects specific biochemical reactions without interfering with other bodily functions. Also, the route of administration is important. It is certainly better, for example, to be able to take a medication by mouth than to use a *parenteral* route—an injection or an intravenous infusion. There are other practical considerations for a pharmaceutical company. Can large quantities be made at a high level of purity? Is it stable when stored? Will new and expensive equipment be needed to produce it? Does the cost of the manufacture exceed the potential for profit?

The final gateway to testing in humans is first to test the product on animals. Again, the ethical questions surrounding the use of animals in human research are outside of the scope of this book. The fact is that as alternatives to using animals are being sought, modern medicine is now absolutely dependent on using animals, both for basic research on the inner workings of disease processes and for initial testing of potential pharmaceuticals to treat those diseases. Using these compounds first in animals, such as mice, rats, and rabbits, reveals how the test substance is absorbed and metabolized (broken down chemically), and whether or not it causes unacceptable side effects or dangerous toxicities.

Once animal safety testing is done, the company then submits detailed results of all of their testing, from the lab bench to animals, in an investigational new drug (IND) application to the FDA, asking for permission to test in humans, in *clinical trials*. If granted, the final, complicated steps begin. All clinical trials must be supervised by a local institutional review board (IRB). An IRB is a panel of scientists, statisticians, ethicists, and nonscientists convened by the institution where the trials are to take place. The IRB is required by federal law to monitor the ethical standards and safety of experiments involving human subjects.

O O O

Before we examine the various stages of clinical trials in which a potential medication is tested on human volunteers, let's look at the basic principles behind accurate, reliable human testing. The modern system of clinical trials evolved first in Britain in the late 1940s, a product of post–World War II medicine. They are an efficient, accurate, systematized way of determining whether or not a particular therapy is safe and effective, at what doses it works best, and what side effects it might cause.

A 1948 test of the antibiotic streptomycin in Britain is often given honors as the first well-known randomized, controlled trial. In a controlled trial, some people are given the investigational drug, while those in a comparable group—the "control" group—are not. Both groups are chosen randomly from all the available volunteers so as not to prejudice the results by deliberately selecting individuals for one group or the other. Then, the effects of the tested versus the nontested control group can be analyzed.

These simple and logical steps were gradually refined into the kind of clinical testing format that we now take for granted. Typically, in a modern, thorough clinical trial—the only legal basis for the FDA to conclude that a new drug has demonstrated "substantial evidence of effectiveness"—the investigators look for subjects who are as similar as possible in ways that can affect the outcome. For example, they must be at the same stage of the disease and be of similar age, weight, and general health. Then the volunteers are randomly assigned to either the control or treatment group.

Despite the best of intentions, there are biases that can affect the scientific validity of a clinical trial. In many cases, for example, during the trial, the treatment group receives the medication being tested, while the control group gets a *placebo*—an ineffective substance that looks like the real thing. In other words, the members of both groups may each get identical-looking small blue pills twice a day. Ideally, the testing is "blinded." If it is *single-blinded* the volunteers do not know if they are receiving the investigational drug or a placebo. In a *double-blinded* trial, neither the subjects nor the investigators have access to that information until the conclusion of the study.

If these rules are followed, any inadvertent skewing of the results is avoided, as can happen in the well-known "placebo effect." The Latin word *placebo* is translated as "I shall please." Due to the well-known but still quite mysterious link between the human brain and the body, the mere notion that one is taking medication that might, for example, relieve pain, can actually have that welcome effect, even though the "medication" is actually quite useless. This placebo effect is very common in RA and underlines the necessity of using carefully controlled studies. In clinical trials people with even severe RA may often feel surprisingly better after a series of placebo treatments, even though trial subjects are not told whether they are in the control or treatment groups.

A good clinical trial requires careful statistical analysis to weed out any unintended biases on the part of investigators and subjects. That takes careful planning in RA studies because judgments about the precise stage of a person's disease and criteria for improvement of that status are not easy to come by. For instance, during the 1990s substantial agreements were reached over standards for clinical research in RA. A basic set of measures has been endorsed by the American

College of Rheumatology (ACR), the European League Against Rheumatism (EULAR), and other organizations. They have designated certain criteria for reporting the responses of people with RA in clinical trials, which has improved the capacity to compare results from various trials.

There is still ongoing discussion about how to improve evaluation of proposed RA medications. Because the primary goal of RA therapy is to improve a person's long-term outcome, many feel that more emphasis needs to be put on following people for extended periods of time with more refined criteria for assessing the status of their disease. Another suggestion is to encourage more testing of people with RA earlier, while they still have little or no joint damage.

The following is the sequence that normally would be followed in typical clinical trials to test any proposed new medication.

Phase I

A small group of healthy volunteers (twenty to eighty) are given the medication in phase I to test its safety and to look for side effects, such as nausea, or pain. The objective here is to determine safety and to find the largest dose that can be tolerated. Valuable information can be gained here about how the drug is changed chemically within the body, how much is absorbed into the blood and organs, and how long it stays in the body. For every one hundred drugs tested in phase I trials, only seventy will go on to phase II.

Phase II

Up to several hundred volunteers, sometimes spread out over a number of different research centers, are chosen for phase II, in which the investigators want to learn whether or not the drug is actually effective against the disease. After phase I, although the drug has an acceptable safety profile and the maximum tolerated dose is now known, more data are collected on safety at this level of testing. At this stage, people with RA are needed as volunteers. Ideally, they must meet strict criteria to be included in a particular study. The subjects may be restricted, for example, to people who have been diagnosed with RA within the previous year, or to those taking methotrexate but not steroids, or to those who have had RA for more than ten years and have failed all available therapies. The point is to test people who share as many characteristics as possible, including the status of their RA and treatment history. After phase II thirty-three of every one hundred drugs tested will move on to phase III.

Phase III

For phase III, the drug is tested on several hundred to several thousand volunteers. Phase I may have taken a few months, and phase II up to two years. The larger scale of phase III may require up to four years. Here, a drug's effectiveness is confirmed, side effects are carefully monitored, and comparisons may be made of commonly used treatments.

If a drug passes phase III testing by proving that is sufficiently safe and effective, the sponsors of the tests can file a new drug application (NDA) with the FDA. This document, which typically runs to one hundred thousand pages or more, is reviewed by the FDA (which often may take more than one year). Once approved by the FDA the new medication is available for physicians to prescribe. However, when a medication is cleared for commercial use, the FDA limits the recommendations for the dose, the formula of the drug, and the precise medical condition that it can be prescribed for, based on the clinical trials for that medication.

If someone wants to alter those conditions, for example, to allow use of the medication in juvenile RA in addition to adult RA, then the medication must go through phase IV testing. These so-called postmarketing studies may be initiated by a pharmaceutical company, may be required by the FDA for a variety of reasons, or may be requested by third parties interested in looking at a drug's application for another stage of the same disease or even another medical condition. Phase IV can go on during the drug approval process, immediately after, or even years later, and take only a few weeks to several years. (However, once a drug is on the market, physicians are free to prescribe it for uses other than the ones for which the FDA has given its approval. This is known as off-label use.)

✪ ✪ ✪

The above "hoops" through which the sponsors of clinical trials must jump are employed in varying degrees in other countries. In 1993, the European Union set in motion a pan-European system for drug approvals. The European Agency for the Evaluation of Medicinal Products (EMEA; www.eudraportal.eudra. org), is the new route for authorizing medicinal products for human and veterinary use. The findings of the EMEA committees, nominated by the member states, are submitted to the European Commission, which makes the final ruling on clearing the product for marketing in all of the fifteen members of the European Union, as well as Iceland and Norway. In Canada, the governmental agency Health Canada (www.hc-sc. gc.ca) has responsibility for approving the sale of any new drug.

Because clinical trials require human volunteers, trials planning includes some serious ethical considerations. First, the volunteers must be given the opportunity for informed consent. This means that they must be given the key facts about the trial before giving written consent. They must, for example, know what research is being done, its goals, what will be done and for how long, what risks might be involved, what benefits might be expected, and understand clearly that they are free to leave the trial at any time.

Other ethical questions have to be considered. For example, can one give volunteers a placebo when at least partially effective treatment for their condition is known? The consensus in the United States, and increasingly abroad, is that fully informed volunteers can agree to take part in a controlled-randomized-double-blinded clinical trial, even when there is effective therapy for their condition, as long as the investigators do not withhold therapy that could alter the volunteers' survival or prevent irreversible injury to them.

If a trial is proceeding, and a major effect—positive or negative—is seen, the trial can be halted. In other words, it would be considered unethical to continue if a treatment was clearly harmful, or if continuing the trial would delay the approval of a clearly effective treatment. In the case of RA trials (as well as in many others) there is the added complexity of answering the question of the long-term effects (which may take years to surface) of a new medication. Clinical trials can answer that question to a point, but although a drug may be approved for use, there is often a period in which physicians are cautious in prescribing a newcomer rather than an old acquaintance.

It's obvious that the transition from an idea to a safe, effective, prescribed medication can be a long and demanding passage. It's also painfully evident that while there has to be great care taken to see to it that drugs are safe as well as effective, the time required to usher a new idea from "bench to bottle" is uncomfortably long. This impatience with the process is felt not only by people who need better treatments as soon as possible, but also by the manufacturers of those treatments, who have taken a multimillion-dollar calculated risk that they will realize a profit within a reasonable period of time.

There are several ways in which this lengthy process gradually is being shortened. One improvement is in the recruitment of people who are willing to participate. All clinical trials have guidelines for eligibility including factors such as age, type of disease, or medical history. Some trials need volunteers with the disease being studied, or healthy people to participate in phase I trials, vaccine studies, or studies on preventive care. There are some advantages to participation, such as gaining access to new treatments, obtaining expert medical care, and helping others by contributing to medical research. Disadvantages to be weighed are the possibilities of experiencing side effects, as well as the requirement of lengthy treatment periods.

Assuming that people want to volunteer (which may include being paid or at least being reimbursed for expenses), the challenge of just rounding up enough people for a valid test is time-consuming. Now, the Internet is beginning to come to the rescue. In February 2000, the National Institutes of Health opened up a Web site (clinicaltrials.gov) listing all clinical trials for serious illnesses. The site also gives useful information on the ins and outs of clinical trials, including questions that people should ask before enrolling.

Another useful site is www.centerwatch.com. This site not only lists trials that are recruiting volunteers, it offers a free notification service that will notify someone when a trial of interest to them is going on in their area. Rheumatology Research International (www.rri.net) is a company that has become a prominent provider in clinical trials site management. Its services include subject recruitment, and one can be put in touch with relevant clinical trials through the site. In addition, Drug Study Central at drugstudycentral.com also assists in finding a specific kind of clinical trial by offering a convenient notification service. In Canada, a useful Clinical Trials Information Service at www.arthritis.ca/clinicaltrials is provided by the Arthritis Society of Canada (www.arthritis.ca).

In addition to speedier recruitment for clinical trials, changes occurring in the technology of medical research promise to streamline drug development. There are new advances in computer-enhanced visualization of molecules, as well as the recent availability of unique instruments that can quickly screen hundreds or even thousands of compounds simultaneously. For example, in looking at the interactions between a cell's proteins and possible therapeutic chemicals— what might have taken many months is now done in a few minutes. The "go/no go" decisions about the practicality of testing a potential medication are being made earlier in the drug development process.

The number of potential targets within the body for drugs is expected to increase dramatically as well, now that science has unraveled so much of the molecular details of human DNA (see chapter 5). The human genome, the full set of genes in each of our cells, carries a code for making about 120,000 to 140,000 different proteins. So far, only about 400 of those proteins are identified targets of drugs used to treat diseases. Many of the others, including the enzymes, cell-surface proteins, and cytokine chemical messengers that operate in RA, will become targets for new medications, either directly or through the regulation of the genes that make them.

This speculation about the future certainly may be encouraging, but what potential new RA treatments are flowing through the "pipeline" now? Which are showing signs that they may soon be available for many with RA for whom the distant future may be of some academic interest, while their present is marked by pain and discouragement?

CHAPTER 10

In the Pipeline

The lengthy passage from dream to drug, from speculation to medication, often begins in a public forum. Reports of preliminary laboratory experiments done in university laboratories, for example, may be published in journals, or perhaps delivered as reports or as poster presentations at scientific conferences. These reports give anyone with an interest in, for example, cancer, AIDS, or RA an opportunity to have an inkling of the new ideas and proposals for novel ways to target those diseases.

This kind of basic research goes on as well in companies whose business it is to develop useful and profitable products. Some publication comes out of this "in-house" research, but other discoveries are understandably held as proprietary, that is, private information. When and if a company deems a potential drug worthy of further testing, and applies to the FDA for permission to enter the drug in human clinical trials, information about those plans becomes public. At various points along this process of moving a drug through the "pipeline" from potential to possible production, a company usually issues press releases about their plans, and more recently, offers relevant information on their Web sites.

Because clinical trials may take years to complete, and only about one-quarter of the products that enter trials are judged worthwhile for further development, unrealistic expectations can sometimes develop about a particular product. Certainly, hopes for anticipated new treatments for RA, as they move for years through the pipeline, have been fulfilled over the past few years (see chapter 8). Other highly touted possibilities have not fared as well. For example, cipemistat (Trocade) appeared to be an impressive candidate for halting or even reversing the destructive effects of the enzyme collagenase, which breaks down cartilage and bone in RA. Unfortunately, Trocade failed to show significant results in clinical trials and was dropped in 2000.

Another interesting approach was tested using interleukin-10. Early clinical trials suggested that administering the anti-inflammatory cytokine chemical interleukin-10 (IL-10), in the form labeled as Tenovil, inhibited the production of the pro-inflammatory cytokines TNF-alpha, interleukin-1 (IL-1) and interleukin-6 (IL-6). Again, further tests did not demonstrate this beneficial effect and Tenovil joined the ranks of potential RA therapies that have been retired from the pipeline.

It is important to remember that both hype and hope are part and parcel of RA research, and pharmaceutical research in general. A company encourages investment by demonstrating that it is investigating substances that show promise as therapeutic agents. Without raising the millions of dollars needed for research and development, the creation, testing, and finally production of new medications would be impossible. And, after all, any investment is a calculated risk.

On the other hand, when news of a possible novel therapy filters out to the public, there is an understandable influx of hope that the potential might become a reality. But because of the long-term testing required before new medications can be prescribed (see chapter 9) one needs to put promises into perspective.

With this introduction in mind, let's take an overview of the current pipeline of potential treatments for RA. None of this information has been gleaned from confidential sources. It is freely available through a variety of resources. The Web sites of pharmaceutical companies are a very useful resource. Their Web site news is usually mirrored by press releases, and eventually many of these are summarized in publications such as the very informative magazine *Arthritis Today*, published by the Arthritis Foundation (www.arthritis.org). For those with some scientific expertise, more technical journal articles and reports of science conferences can be obtained in libraries or through the Internet at sites such as PubMed at www.ncbi.nlm.nih.gov/PubMed. These sources and many others are outlined in the appendix.

The following account encompasses the testing of (1) potential therapies that appear close to completion, (2) those that are further back in the process, and (3) intriguing new approaches to striking back at RA from different directions through methods yet to face the rigors of clinical trials. All of these therapies center around our current, only partial understanding of the RA disease process (Fig. 14). Each step along the series of interactions of cells and chemicals that leads to and sustains the inflammation, swelling, pain, and damage of RA offers a potential target for slowing down the process, easing the pain, and perhaps even helping to stop it altogether.

Blocking TNF-alpha

In chapter 8 we saw how two new medications, Enbrel and Remicade, block the inflammatory chemical TNF-alpha (Fig. 14). The pharmaceutical company BASF Pharma, Ludwigshafen, Germany (www.basf-pharma.com), is optimistic about D2E7, its antibody against TNF-alpha, developed in collaboration with Cambridge Antibody Technology, Cambridgeshire, U.K. (www.

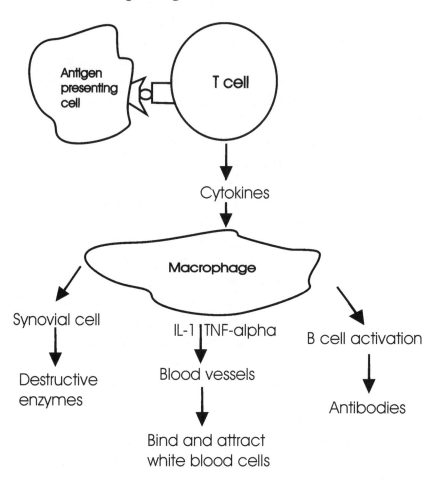

Fig. 14. A generalized scheme of the inflammatory process seen in RA. Antigens (whose identity is not yet known) activate T cells and set off a cascade of events marked by release of chemical messages, including IL-1 and TNF-alpha, that drives inflammation.

cambridgeantibody.com). BASF Pharma began enrolling volunteers for phase III clinical trials in mid-2000. This antibody has so far shown the ability to reduce joint inflammation and relieve the signs and symptoms of RA by "mopping up" excess TNF-alpha. There is evidence from X-ray analysis that it can also slow down the progression of RA damage, a very desirable effect.

According to BASF Pharma, D2E7 lasts longer after injection, so it can be administered once per week instead of the twice-weekly injections for Enbrel, which means it could turn out to be more convenient and less expensive. Because it is a human antibody it stimulates fewer allergic and injection site reactions. An advantage claimed over Remicade is that, unlike with Remicade, it is not necessary to give D2E7 in conjunction with methotrexate.

CellTech Chiroscience, Berkshire, U.K. (www.celltech.co.uk), also has a chemically modified TNF-alpha antibody, CDP 870, which went into phase II testing in 2000. In earlier studies, which lasted for an eight-week period, a single intravenous infusion of CDP870 produced a rapid and long-lasting improvement in people with active RA, including 70 to 80 percent reductions in the number of tender joints, and 60 to 70 percent reductions in swollen joints.

Serono, Geneva, Switzerland (www.serono.com), is developing its own anti-TNF-alpha approach. Serono's product, rTBP-1, is a soluble receptor for TNF-alpha that can latch onto that cytokine and keep it from coming in contact with other cells and triggering inflammation. Phase II trials began in 2000.

Another soluble TNF-alpha receptor, sTNF-R1, was in phase II clinical trials as well, under the auspices of Amgen, Inc., Thousand Oaks, California (www.amgen.com).

Meanwhile, Isis Pharmaceuticals, Carlsbad, California (www.isip.com), planned on starting phase I/II clinical trials in late 2000–2001 with its unique TNF-alpha blocker, ISIS 104838. This is neither an antibody nor a soluble receptor like the above compounds; it is a laboratory-synthesized antisense molecule. This means that this oral medication will, if early indications are predictive, enter the joints, move into cells there, and interfere with the messages coming from the genes in those cells responsible for making the TNF-alpha molecules. The message from the genes no longer "makes sense" and the cells cannot make TNF-alpha, so the amount of this inflammatory substance will be reduced.

Our list of anti-TNF-alpha techniques includes an unusual, nontoxic method of whole-body hyperthermia that has been shown at the University of Wisconsin, Madison, Wisconsin (www.wisc.edu), to induce a rise in levels of soluble TNF-receptor. When volunteers were heated to 41.8° Celsius (107.2° Fahrenheit) for sixty minutes, the levels of this substance, which the body makes as a natural antidote to rising levels of TNF-alpha, increased measurably. In RA, the natural levels of TNF receptor are not enough to combat the effects of the disease, and this treatment is aimed at possibly inducing remission in people with active RA. In 2000, scientists at the university began recruiting volunteers for phase I trials.

Blocking IL-1

The cytokine chemical interleukin-1 (IL-1), along with TNF-alpha, is considered to be central to the inflammatory and destructive processes of RA (Fig. 14). In fact, IL-1 can induce the production of TNF-alpha, and vice versa. Included among the nasty effects of IL-1 are an increase in COX-2, the enzyme that enhances inflammation (and is the target of the new anti-inflammatory drug Celebrex, described in chapter 8). IL-1 also stimulates the production of molecules that line the blood vessels and grab onto passing white blood cells, luring them to enter the irritated tissues and contribute to the inflammation. This cytokine also contributes to the eventual breakdown of bone tissue in the joints. Its actions go beyond the joints and contribute to more general reactions such as loss of appetite and fatigue. Again, it's important to remember that all these effects of this cytokine and others released by the body's immune system are part of a natural, complex set of events designed to defend against injury and infection. When these responses are excessive and prolonged, as in the case of RA, they provoke and maintain inflammatory disease.

The pivotal role played by IL-1 in RA makes it a natural target for therapies directed at reversing its destructive effects. But how can one interfere with its activities? Just as we described in the case TNF-alpha, the other major inflammatory cytokine, IL-1 acts by being recognized by special receptors on cell surfaces. Those receptors, which are proteins, will act as a lock into which the IL-1 molecule easily fits. Once this meeting takes place, a cascade of reactions is set off inside the cell, genes are turned on, and the cell can then make substances that contribute to inflammation, such as destructive enzymes.

As it turns out, the body makes another slightly different form of IL-1, which also can fit the receptor locks. This form is interleukin-1 receptor antagonist (IL-1ra). The crucial difference between IL-1 and IL-1ra is that when IL-1ra fits into the receptors, the cascade of reactions does not take place inside the cell. In other words, IL-1ra is a natural control the body uses to balance the inflammatory effects of IL-1. It competes for the receptor sites sought out by IL-1. It's as though the IL-1 receptor sites were reserved parking spots. The IL-1ra molecules park there instead, leaving nowhere for the IL-1 molecules to park and get on with their work of inflammation. However, it takes relatively high concentrations of IL-1ra to counteract the effects of IL-1. Studies have shown that the natural levels of IL-1ra in people with RA are not sufficient to control the disease.

We saw in chapter 5 that preliminary tests in humans showed that genes for making IL-1ra can be put into human joints, and further study is in progress. At this point, however, a different approach is very near the final stages of FDA approval. Amgen, Inc., Thousand Oaks, California (www.amgen.com), the same company that is testing a TNF-alpha receptor (see above), has developed a promising RA therapy using IL-1ra.

The medication, anakinra (Kineret), will probably soon become the first of a new class of RA medications. It is a "recombinant" form of human IL-1ra, which means that scientists at Amgen have used the human gene that makes IL-1ra and put the gene into batches of cells growing in the laboratory. The cells dutifully follow the instructions of the gene and make IL-1ra, offering an ample supply for medical use. This is an example of *genetic engineeering.*

Extensive clinical trials of injections of this recombinant human IL-1ra have shown it to be an effective treatment that can both reduce inflammation and slow bone and cartilage destruction. Interestingly, when the IL-1ra is used in conjunction with the soluble TNF-alpha receptor, described earlier in this chapter and also made by Amgen, the beneficial effects are greater than when either is used alone.

A different strategy for foiling the IL-1 molecules is employed by using a soluble form of a receptor for IL-1. The use of this receptor is in the early stages of development at the Immunex Corporation, Seattle, Washington (www.immunex.com). In its soluble form, the receptor, ordinarily on cell surfaces, can latch onto IL-1 and prevent it from attaching to cells and causing trouble.

Yet another way to prevent trouble caused by IL-1 is to cut down on its production in the first place. The building blocks of IL-1 molecules that exist inside the cells (such as macrophages, Fig. 14) that produce it cannot be released from those cells in the active, inflammatory form unless they are acted on by an enzyme known as ICE. Vertex Pharmaceuticals, Inc., Cambridge, Massachusetts (www.vpharm.com), in collaboration with Aventis, Strasbourg, France (www.aventis.com), discovered and developed a substance that inhibits the activity of the ICE enzyme. They first analyzed the three-dimensional structure of ICE, laying the foundation for designing molecules that could bind to it and prevent it from functioning.

Their product VX-740, in a convenient oral form, was in phase II clinical trials in 2000. This is the only example of this unique approach to RA therapy.

In addition to VX-740, Vertex and Aventis have entered another product, VX-745, into phase II clinical trials. VX-745 takes aim at another enzyme, a member of a group of molecules called MAP enzymes. This particular enzyme target plays a vital role in the production of not only IL-1, but also TNF-alpha and another inflammatory cytokine interleukin-6 (IL-6).

Blocking IL-2

Tacrolimus (Prograf FK506), a powerful drug that is useful in organ and bone marrow transplants, is being tested against RA. Tacrolimus has been shown to inhibit the proinflammatory cytokines IL-2 (and IL-6, as well as slow down the production of COX-2, the target of the newer RA anti-inflammatories). A small-scale phase II clinical trial with twelve subjects with severe, active RA showed that although five subjects left the trial with side effects, seven had significant relief. In 1999, Fujisawa Healthcare, Deerfield, Illinois (www.fujisawausa. com), began large-scale phase III clinical trials of Tacrolimus at about fifty testing centers.

Vaccines

In April 1999, the U.S. Institute of Medicine (IOM; www.iom. edu), an advisor to the federal government on scientific and technological matters, published the the results of their four-year effort to study priorities for vaccine development. In the top ranks of those priorities, based on the potential for reducing expenses and increasing quality of life, was a vaccine for RA.

Most people tend to think of vaccines as injections that we are given when we are vaccinated against diseases like tetanus, whooping cough, measles, or polio. In a wider sense, a vaccine can be any inoculation that can confer immunity against a specific disease. In the case of the diseases just mentioned and others, injecting either entire bacteria or viruses that have been rendered harmless, or even just parts of those organisms that can act as antigens, sets off an immune response in the body that stimulates the production of antibodies aimed directly at those specific disease-causing organisms, rendering us immune to them. This lifesaving immunity may be permanent or require an occasional reinoculation, such as a tetanus "booster."

In terms of RA, there are several ways in which scientists are using vaccines not to stimulate an antibody response to bacteria or viruses, but to interfere with particular steps in the RA disease process. Corixa Corp., Seattle, Washington (www. corixa.com), went through successful phase II clinical trial testing in 2000 with its innovative AnervaX.RA vaccine. This is a laboratory-synthesized small protein fragment, based on part of a protein genetically linked to RA. In other words, this vaccine is identical to part of a protein shared by many people with RA. In autoimmune diseases like RA, the immune system unfortunately recognizes components of the body's own cells and tissues as antigens, that is, dangerous foreign substances, and turns the immune system against them.

These self-antigen components (we are not sure yet of their exact identity) are picked up by cells like the macrophages represented in figure 14, and "presented" to T cells. As we described in some detail in chapter 4, this presentation of the antigens has to be made by attaching the antigens to special protein holders, the MHC molecules on the antigen-presenting cells. This is the site that the AnervaX.RA vaccine affects. It stimulates the production of antibodies that block that presentation of self-antigens to the T cells (Fig. 14) and helps to prevent progression of the disease.

Corixa, in collaboration with NV Organon, Oss, the Netherlands (www.organon.com), is developing another related drug that demonstrated good results against RA in phase I/II clinical trials that were completed in late 2000. It is not a vaccine, but we will describe its action here for convenience. It is AnergiX.RA, which is a mix of some of those MHC "protein holders" just described, attached to a protein fragment from human cartilage. This fragment is thought to be at least one of the body's antigens that T cells react against in RA. Giving the cartilage molecules neatly held in the MHC holders that the T cells are accustomed to latching onto, and thereby becoming activated to cause inflammation, could plug up the receptors on the T cells with AnergiX.RA, which would not activate the T cells, but instead put them out of commission.

The Immune Response Corporation, Carlsbad, California (www.imnr.com), is aiming its vaccine against the other member of the antigen-presenting cell and the T cell pair. The basis for their decision to strike at the T cells is the discovery that in the human immune system there are literally millions of T cell types, each with a slightly different form of T cell receptor (TCR). The TCR is the protein that joins with the antigen held out to it by the antigen-presenting cell (Fig. 14).

This means that in rheumatoid arthritis, when the antigens that set off the disease are presented to T cells, those particular T cells begin to multiply wildly and build up a large population of identical, activated T cells that can fan the flames of RA. If one could eliminate those particular activated populations of T cells, then the disease might be stopped. Following this principle, researchers isolated T cells from joint tissues of people with RA and identified a small set of TCR protein fragments that seem to be often typical of arthritic but not normal tissues.

They then made a vaccine preparation using a mixture of three of these protein fragments, and injected this vaccine, IR501, into volunteers in phase I/II clinical trials with encouraging results. What seems to be happening is that the vaccine stimulates the immune system to make antibodies against those injected protein fragments. Because those fragments are identical to parts of the protein receptors on the trouble-making T cells, the antibodies grab onto those T cell receptors and block them from doing any further harm. In other words, this may be a way to delete, suppress, or inactivate the harmful T cell types from the immune system of a person with RA by a few simple injections. That would leave all the other T cell types available to operate the normal defenses of the body. This vaccine method was headed for phase III clinical trials in 2000.

More Antibodies

Those troublesome T cells have become a favorite target for potential RA therapies. Another way to get at them, in addition to the vaccines just discussed, is to fashion antibodies directed at a specific parts of the T cells that are most active in RA. On at least 60 percent of those kind of T cells there is an important protein, CD4, that aids in the binding of the T cells and the antigen-presenting cells (Fig. 14). It seems logical to try to block the CD4's ability to help the T cells become activated. Early attempts to use antibodies made in mice against CD4 were promising, but the effects were short-lived, and because the antibodies were from animals, the human subjects, ironically, formed antibodies against the CD4 antibodies.

Advances in antibody technology have made it possible to make fully human monoclonal antibodies (Mabs), directed against specific, unique antigens. (In fact, by 2001 more than one-quarter of all the biotechnology drugs in development for many different diseases were Mabs, and over two hundred Mabs were in clinical trials). Medarex, Inc., Princeton, New Jersey (www.medarex.com), had two Mabs directed against CD4 on the T cells in people with RA—MDX-33 and MDX-24—in phase II clinical trials in 2000. In that same year, IDEC Pharmaceuticals, San Diego, California (www.idecpharm.com), entered phase II clinical trials with its candidate for anti-CD4 therapy in the form of Clenoliximab (IDEC-151). (While not yet in clinical trials, IDEC hopes to initiate trials on its antibodies against MIF, an immune system chemical that attracts macrophages, those antigen-presenting cells that assist in inflammation.)

Other proinflammatory cytokines besides IL-1 and TNF-alpha have received some attention as targets to attack with antibodies. One that entered phase I clinical trials in 2000 as a target was interleukin-12 (IL-12). BASF Pharma (mentioned earlier as the developer of the TNF-alpha antibody), in collaboration with Genetics Institute, Cambridge, Massachusetts (www.genetics.com), have produced a fully human antibody, J695, which snares IL-12 molecules and prevents them from going about their inflammatory business.

A unique category of antibody targets, the *complement* system, joined the ranks of those in phase II clinical trials in 2000. The complement system is a group of normally well-behaved proteins that are very abundant in human blood. When signaled by an infection, injury, or the formation of antigen-antibody complexes such as happens in RA, a cascade of chemical reactions is set off within that collection of complement proteins, resulting in forms of proteins that aid in inflammation. This is a normal, protective series of reactions, but if there is constant stimulus of this complement system, as in RA, the inflammation is painfully inappropriate.

Alexion Pharmaceuticals, New Haven, Connecticut (www.alexionpharmaceuticals.com), has designed a promising monoclonal antibody that selectively blocks one of the important intermediates in the cascade of complement reactions. The drug, 5G1.1, was in phase II clinical trials in 2000.

Antibodies Against B Cells

Dr. Jonathan Edwards and his colleagues at the Centre for Rheumatology, University College, London, have developed the hypothesis that RA is caused by certain B cells. By chance, these cells make autoantibodies, that is, antibodies against the person's own tissues. The immune system ordinarily would destroy these B cells, but in rare cases these unusual antibodies escape destruction and actually set up a vicious cycle that triggers the production of many copies of themselves, resulting in the self-sustained attack on joints and tissues seen in RA.

If this hypothesis is correct, it would seem logical that wiping out the B cells might elminate the very cause of RA. Because a depletion of B cells is not life threatening, and the B cell population gradually reestablishes itself after several months, the assumption is that the new B cell population would be unlikely to include any cells that make the unusual antibodies that lead to RA.

Edwards and coworkers began preliminary trials in 1998 with five people suffering from severe RA, and for whom no treatments had been effective. The volunteers were given rituximab (Mabthera), a monoclonal antibody that destroys B cells, as well as steroids and an immunosuppresive drug. Eighteen months later the researchers could report that these five volunteers " . . . now only have some residual pain from the damage already done. They have returned to a more or less normal life. . . . "

Fifteen more people with severe RA underwent the same procedure. By late 2000, only two of the twenty treated had shown no benefits, and although several of the responders relapsed, they achieved significant relief after another round of antibody treatment. Much more extensive clinical trials involving 160 people with RA in Europe, Australia, and Canada are planned for 2001–2002. This unique approach is explained and updated by Professor Edwards at (www.ucl. ac.uk/ ~ regfjxe).

Other Avenues

Experiments over a number of years have demonstrated clearly that immunity to certain antigens can be induced by feeding animals with samples of those antigens. Of particular interest in this demonstration of *oral tolerance* has been the effective use of collagen, a cartilage protein, in animals with experimentally induced arthritis similar to RA. Collagen type II (CII), which is a major component of joint cartilage, can suppress arthritis in several different animal species. The theory behind the effect is that if the animal is fed proteins similar to the ones being attacked by the disease, the immune system may be fooled into treating the proteins with the same respect that it gives food molecules. After all, we are constantly eating substances that our immune systems would regard as dangerous antigens if they were injected, but which are spared if they are absorbed from the gastrointestinal tract. However, we really do not yet understand how oral tolerance works, and whether or not we can harness it for therapeutic purposes.

This idea of oral tolerance induction, while intriguing, has not had the hoped-for results in clinical trials so far. The results up to now suggest that oral collagen may produce some benefit in a minority of people. A large-scale, multicenter, phase II trial of oral type II collagen, with an anticipated completion date of August, 2002, is underway under the direction of the University of Tennessee, Memphis (www.utmem.edu), and Vanderbilt University Medical Center (www.mc.vanderbilt.edu).

A unique approach to RA therapy is being taken by Protein Therapeutics, Tucson, Arizona, affiliated with Research Corporation Technologies (RCT), also in Tucson (www.rctech.com). One hypothesis behind the partial success of their phase I/II clinical trials proposed therapy for RA is the idea that oral administration of the antibody fraction of human blood may give people with RA new antibodies that can neutralize viral or bacterial disease-associated antigens, not allowing them to trigger an autoimmune response. The immunoglobulin fraction of human blood, often referred to as gamma globulin, pooled from healthy individuals, has been used for years as a quick, convenient source of antibodies for people exposed to infectious diseases such as measles or hepatitis. In late 2000, the companies were planning an extensive phase III trial in hopes of obtaining FDA approval for their oral immunoglobulin preparation, IgPO, in this unique procedure.

Thalidomide, the infamous sedative that was banned after it caused serious birth defects and malformations in ten thousand babies worldwide in the 1950s, has a new life. In 1998 the FDA approved thalidomide for, of all things, a painful form of leprosy, as well as for multiple myeloma, a cancer of the bone marrow. Careful studies on the action of thalidomide have revealed that it can block the growth of blood vessels and also decrease levels of TNF-alpha.

Because of thalidomide's mode of action, Celgene Corporation, Warren, New Jersey (www.celgene.com), a leader in thalidomide research, has examined ways in which this drug might be useful in the fight against RA. Because of its disturbing past and the fact that it is a toxic substance that must be used with care, particularly with women of child-bearing age, Celgene has been creating forms of thalidomide that differ from the original molecule. It turns out that several of these new molecules can inhibit COX-2, the proinflammatory enzyme blocked by the new anti-inflammatory Celebrex (see chapter 8). Celgene hopes to find safe and effective derivatives of thalidomide for RA therapy.

Ligand Pharmaceuticals, Inc., San Diego, California (www.ligand.com), is working toward possible clinical trials with its ONTAK molecule. This medication is already approved for use in a particular form of cancer in which malignant cells have a protein receptor on their surface for interleukin-2 (IL-2), a receptor that is usually found on activated T cells, and some other immune system cells. This medication attaches itself to the IL-2 receptors on the cell surface and causes the cells to die. It seems logical that this ability to hit at inflammatory T cells might allow the use of ONTAK in RA.

Another substance, infamous in its own right, was reported in late 2000 to have a beneficial impact on mice with a rheumatoid arthritis–like disease. An extract of marijuana, cannabidiol (which does not induce a "high" in consumers), was given to the animals, who responded by having significantly fewer arthritic symptoms, and less damage to their joints (pardon the expression). Dr. Marc Feldmann, a prominent arthritis researcher and principal author of the report suggested that the time is ripe to do clinical trials with human subjects.

Somewhat earlier that same year, the FDA paved the way for related trials when they approved Atlantic Technology Ventures' (ATV) IND application for CT3, a synthetic marijuana derivative. ATV, New York, New York (www.atlan.com), hopes that CT3 will offer relief from pain and inflammation and can become a safe alternative to NSAIDs (see chapter 7), which can have sometimes serious gastrointestinal side effects. A phase I trial in Europe began in late 2000 under the direction of the Aster Clinical Research Center (www.aster-cephac.fr) in Paris. It was expected to provide useful results for an anticipated phase I trial in the United States.

Strange as it may seem, nitric oxide (NO), a colorless gas that is a component of automobile exhaust, is now known to be an important biological molecule in our bodies. It is made by many cells, including those lining our blood vessels, cartilage cells, and immune system cells like macrophages. Scientists are still trying to track down all of the many effects that this highly reactive gas has in our cells and tissues. Like many other body substances, the amount is important—a little may be good, and too much may cause trouble. NO can have both anti- and proinflammatory effects. It plays a role in regulating the expansion of blood vessel walls as well.

NicOx S.A., Sophia-Antipolis, France (www. nicox.com), is aiming at using the ability of NO to counteract some of the negative gastrointestinal effects of NSAIDs, like ibuprofen or aspirin (see chapter 7). Their experimental medications are called NO-NSAIDs, and combine a conventional nonsteroidal compound with a component that releases small amounts of NO, aimed at preventing ulceration and bleeding.

In the human body, certain NO levels are also linked to destructive conditions, such as a rise in inflammatory prostaglandins. For example, there is increased production of NO in inflamed cartilage. Research continues on the exact role of NO in the immune system, and on finding the best way to use this versatile and important substance in controlling RA.

Angiogenesis, the controlled growth of new blood vessels, is a natural, common process in the human body as it grows and develops. There are situations, however, in which it would very useful to prevent new vessels from forming. This is particularly true in the case of cancerous tumors, which need a rich blood supply. In RA, the inflamed synovium, the lining of the joint, is only able to grow into the pannus, that large, invasive, destructive tissue mass (see chapter 3), by recruiting new blood vessels to supply it nutrition and inflammatory cells.

There is as yet no drug on the market to inhibit the angiogenesis in RA, but considerable progress has been made in research on antiangiogenesis therapies to control tumor growth. It is uncertain which new substance, out of the many known inhibitors of angiogenesis, will prove to be best fitted to treat RA as well as cancer. Several interesting possibilities are being looked at by Chris Storgard and colleagues at the Scripps Research Institute, La Jolla, California (www.scripps. edu). They have used an inhibitor of *integrin*, which is a molecule that encourages angiogenesis, to reduce the severity of RA-like symptoms in rabbits. This inhibitor is expected eventually to enter clinical trials. The Scripps group is also working on preclinical investigations of a monoclonal antibody against integrin in collaboration with Medimmune, Inc., Gaithersburg, Maryland (www.medimmune. com).

The natural biological process of apoptosis is also under intense investigation for a variety of diseases, including RA. Apoptosis is usually a normal, controlled cell death that the body uses for eliminating unwanted, damaged, or superfluous cells. However, the process can go awry as in cancer, in which the mechanisms for getting rid of cells are not sufficient. Likewise, in RA, the body is unable to control the growth of the erosive pannus, the tumorlike growth in the joints. In terms of RA therapies, numerous laboratories are making progress in taking apart the complicated reactions of apoptosis to find ways of either inducing apoptosis to get rid of, for example, inflammatory T cells, or to kill off dividing cells in the pannus.

MCP is a cytokine chemical produced by cells in the lining of rheumatoid joints, in response to those troublemaking cytokines IL-1 and TNF-alpha. MCP is a powerful attractant for inflammatory cells like macrophages. In August 2000, a Canadian research team headed by Chris Overall at the University of British Columbia Faculty of Dentistry, Vancouver, British Columbia (www.dentistry.ubc.ca), discovered that a natural form of MCP, called MCP-3, can halt the flow of the inflammatory cells. It appears that in RA this natural control may malfunction, leading to continuous inflammation. They are studying the details of this system, with the aim of designing new anti-inflammatory drugs.

Cytokines that play a role in attracting white blood cells to a site where they are needed to react against infection or injury are referred to as *chemokines*. Because each of these attractants is a protein, each has a gene responsible for its synthesis in the body. Nathan Karin and colleagues from Technion-Israel Institute of Technology, Haifa, Israel (www. technion.ac.il), have reported that injecting into rats DNA that carried the genetic code for making four of these cytokines protected the mice against developing autoimmune arthritis. These are called naked DNA vaccines.

They showed that, although rats with the disease did make antibodies against these chemokines, the antibodies could not stop the disease from progressing. However, administering the DNA vaccines increased the antibody production and inhibited RA-like arthritis in development and progression, even in rats that already had the disease. This work, reported in late 2000, showed that the mice generated antibodies against each of the chemokines when those antibodies were needed. The researchers are aiming at refining this method to fashion an ideal DNA vaccine that will suppress autoimmunity without seriously inhibiting the day-to-day need for a protective immune system. Clinical trials are expected within several years.

✪ ✪ ✪

As you can see from this survey of current pharmaceutical research, the rich variety of potential therapies for RA that are passing through the "pipeline" leading from possibility to reality must undergo careful scrutiny for safety and effectiveness. Any product that eventually is allowed to join the fight against RA must meet rigorous standards—which can be time-consuming. But while this pipeline of promise is not filled to capacity, and some future therapies introduced in this chapter may be several years away from approval, others are nearly ready. In addition, our rapidly accumulating insights about the human immune system and how RA uses that system to inflict damage and suffering, is leading researchers to pin-point new, precise targets for treatments.

We can say with certainty that the pipeline, now passing judgment on a wide spectrum of novel therapies for RA, will continue to flow with increasing numbers of exciting new pos-sibilities for controlling and even preventing the pain and pro-gression of this disease that has interfered in the lives of so many of us. This and other chapters, as well as the appendix to this book, lists numerous Web sites to help you keep track of announcements about the latest breakthroughs, and the latest treatments. The World Wide Web—accessible through your own computer, or that of a friend, family member, or the local public library—has become the premier portal for infor-mation. Companies, including the ones listed in this chapter, continue to update their Web sites as therapies evolve, and arthritis-centered sites are quick to inform you about the latest RA news.

Afterword

Rheumatoid arthritis is a frustrating disease. While the disease in all people with RA has much in common, the condition may express itself in many different degrees of intensity, flares, and remissions. Medications that may bring relief to some individuals are of little help to others. Even useful medications may lose their effectiveness over time. But this disease, which profoundly affects the lives of so many millions of people, is now under intense scrutiny by researchers who have insights into autoimmunity as well as new tools, unavailable only a few years ago, to investigate and manipulate the human immune system.

There was a palpable sense of optimism among the 460 researchers and physicians who convened in late February 2000 in Chicago at the first ever Clinical Update on New Therapies for the Rheumatic Diseases sponsored by the American College of Rheumatology. New breakthroughs and new therapies, as well as the ways in which these therapies are being applied, mark the beginnings of a new era of unprecedented hope for people with RA.

While a little knowledge is a dangerous thing, no knowledge at all is even worse. Even better is to know the basic vocabulary of RA and its treatment, and to have some insight into the inner workings of our immune system in health and in disease. It is a great advantage as well to appreciate the rationale behind the use of particular medications, and to better understand the treatment choices that are available. My intention has been to introduce the interested reader to what we now know about RA, and to offer encouragement and hope by reviewing the exciting, ongoing progress in understanding and treating this disease.

As I emphasized in the preface, this book is not intended as specific medical advice. Rather, I want to support and encourage the crucially important physician-client relationship by helping people to become better-informed advocates as partners with their physicians in the management of their disease. Early diagnosis and careful treatment, usually with a combination of therapies, many of which have only become available in the last several years, combined with the knowledge that there is a pipeline filling with intriguing possibilities for even more effective treatments, is encouraging for us all.

We shall continue to take advantage of the new and emerging opportunities for treatment of RA, and have good reasons to anticipate the arrival of ever more effective, precisely targeted pharmaceuticals that will silence the cells and chemical messages whose secrets are only now being revealed.

And we shall conquer this disease . . .

APPENDIX

The Inflammation Superhighway

The Internet is an extraordinary, worldwide system of millions of virtually interconnected computers. It offers a unique opportunity to obtain useful information, exchange ideas, and have access to knowledge on a previously unimagined scale. The World Wide Web is a communication system that allows easy access to the Internet. Because literally anyone can set up a Web site, it's important, particularly in the case of medical information, to use sources whose accuracy can be trusted.

While most comprehensive Web sites dedicated to a particular subject have some unique features, they also offer links to many informative, related sites. In addition to the many sites already listed in this book, the following are major Web sites that offer a wide variety of useful information about RA, and include links to many other helpful sources. Many of these sites offer frequent updates on breaking news in research and treatment, message boards where one can post questions or comments and get feedback, or live "chat rooms" where one can enter into discussions online. The best way to learn about the individual features of these Web sites is to visit them and see what they have to offer.

GOOD STARTING POINTS

These include sites specializing in arthritis, as well as sites of organizations dedicated to arthritis. All contain many references to RA.

Arthritis Foundation
www.arthritis.org

American Autoimmune Related Diseases Association
www.aarda.org

Arthritis Research Campaign
www.arc.org.uk

American College of Rheumatology
www.rheumatology.org

Arthritis Canada
www.arthritis.ca

Johns Hopkins Arthritis
www.hopkins-arthritis.com

About.com Guide to Arthritis
arthritis.about.com

RA Information Network
www.healthtalk.com/rain/rainindex.html

drdoc on-line
www.arthritis.co.za

Arthritis Resource Center
www.healingwell.com/arthritis

Arthritis Insight
arthritisinsight.com

Arthritis National Research Foundation
www.curearthritis.org

**National Institute of Arthritis and
Musculoskeletal and Skin Diseases**
www.nih.gov/niams

Asia Pacific League of Associations for Rheumatology
www.ilar.org

Arthritis.com
www.arthritis.com

JUVENILE RHEUMATOID ARTHRITIS

JRA World
www.jraworld.arthritisinsight.com

Pediatric Rheumatology Home Page
www.goldscout.com

HealthlinkUSA
www.healthlinkusa.com/399.html

MEDICAL SITES WITH RA INFORMATION

Medem
www.medem.com

Medscape
rheumatology.medscape.com

PubMed
www.ncbi.nlm.nih.gov/PubMed

BioMedNet
www.bmn.com

WebMD
www.webmd.com

PDR's Getting Well Network
www.gettingwell.com

Yahoo! Health
health.yahoo.com

iVillage AllHealth
www.allhealth.com

Discovery Health
www.discoveryhealth.com

DRUG INFORMATION

Pharmaceutical Information Network
www.pharminfo. com

Medscape
promini.medscape.com/drugdb/search.asp

NEWSGROUPS AND DISCUSSION GROUPS

These are message boards where one can post questions or comments so that users can respond. Find newsgroups at:

www.dejanews.com

www.Emissary.Net/arthritis

Glossary

ACTIVATION Stimulation of cells to make them active, e.g., T cells coming in contact with presented antigens will activate the T cells.

ALLOGENEIC A bone marrow transplant in which the donor of the marrow is a different person from the recipient.

AMINO ACID The building block of proteins. There are twenty different amino acids.

ANGIOGENESIS The formation of new blood vessels.

ANKYLOSING SPONDYLITIS Rheumatoid inflammation of one or more vertebrae.

ANTIBIOTIC A substance produced by an organism that can kill or prevent the growth of other organisms, e.g., penicillin, which is made by fungi.

ANTIBODY   A protein made by a B cell. It can recognize and attach to a specific site on an antigen, rendering it harmless.

ANTIGEN   A substance, often a protein, that induces the production of antibodies.

ANTIGEN PRESENTING CELL (APC)   A cell such as a macrophage that can present antigens to lymphocytes and help to activate the lymphocytes.

APHERESIS   Separating blood into its components.

APOPTOSIS   Cell death that is a natural process.

ARTHRITIS   Inflammation of a joint, usually accompanied by pain and swelling.

AUTOIMMUNE DISEASE   Disease in which one's immune system attacks part of the body.

AUTOLOGOUS   A bone marrow transplant in which a person receives his/her own marrow, removed at an earlier date.

B CELL   White blood cells (leukocytes) that produce antibodies.

B CELL RECEPTOR   A protein on the surface of a B cell that recognizes and can attach to a specific protein.

BIOCHEMICAL   Referring to chemicals that make up living organisms.

BIOLOGIC THERAPY   Therapy based on the use of materials derived from living organisms.

BONE MARROW   The soft material filling the cavities inside bones—the site of blood cell formation.

BONE MARROW TRANSPLANT   The transfer of bone marrow from a donor to a recipient.

BURSA   A sac, in the vicinity of joints, lined with a synovial membrane.

BURSITIS   Inflammation of a bursa.

C-REACTIVE PROTEIN   A protein produced by the liver, and present at elevated levels in RA.

CARTILAGE   A tissue composed of cells embedded in a firm, dense protein substance. One site of cartilage is at the ends of bones where they come together at the joints.

CAPILLARIES   The smallest blood vessels. Fluid and sometimes cells can leave capillaries and enter tissues.

CELL   The smallest organized unit of living matter, e.g., blood cells or skin cells. Each is surrounded by a thin cell membrane.

CELL MEMBRANE   A thin membrane of proteins and fats surrounding each living cell.

CHEMOKINE   Chemical produced by certain cells that helps attract white blood cells to sites of inflammation.

CHONDROITIN SULFATE   One of the chemicals present in cartilage.

CHROMOSOME   A large, coiled DNA molecule, with attached proteins, and containing genes. Humans have forty-six chromosomes in each cell—twenty-three inherited from the mother, and twenty-three from the father.

CLINICAL TRIALS   Organized tests of potential medical treatments using human volunteers.

COLLAGEN   The major protein in cartilage.

COLLAGEN-INDUCED ARTHRITIS (CIA)   A type of arthritis resembling RA induced in animals.

CONNECTIVE TISSUE   A type of tissue that supports and connects structures of the body, e.g., bone, cartilage.

COMPLEMENT   A group of blood proteins involved in inflammation. The complement system can be activated by interaction with antibodies.

CO-RECEPTOR   Proteins on the surface of B or T cells that assist in the binding to other cells.

CORTISONE   A hormone from the outer layer of the adrenal gland. It can also be prepared synthetically.

COX An enzyme, cyclooxygenase, found in two forms, COX-1 and COX-2.

COX-1 An enzyme made by many tissues of the body where it is active in normal cellular functions.

COX-2 An enzyme made in large amounts during inflammation.

CROHN'S DISEASE An inflammatory bowel disease affecting the small intestine.

CYTOKINES Molecules that cells make in order to communicate with other cells.

CYTOTOXIC A substance poisonous to cells.

COLLAGEN TYPE II A protein found in cartilage. When injected into animals it can cause an RA-like inflammation.

DMARD A disease-modifying antirheumatic drug. DMARDS are used in an attempt to slow the progression of RA.

DNA Deoxyribonucleic acid—the chemical out of which our genes are made.

DEGENERATIVE JOINT DISEASE Another term for osteoarthritis.

DENDRITIC CELL A type of cell in tissues that picks up antigens and then goes to the lymphatic tissues where it presents the antigens to T cells.

DOUBLE-BLINDED   A type of clinical trial in which neither the researchers nor the subjects know what treatment, if any, the subjects are receiving, in order to eliminate bias. At the end of the trial that information is revealed to allow analysis.

EMBRYONIC STEM CELLS   Stem cells derived from the inner mass of cells in a young embryo.

ENZYMES   Proteins that assist in chemical reactions.

ERYTHROCYTE SEDIMENTATION RATE   A laboratory test measuring the rate at which the erythrocytes (red blood cells) settle out in a tube. The rate is faster in active RA. Also called the *sed rate*.

FIBROMYALGIA   A syndrome of pervasive musculoskeletal pain, localized tenderness, and fatigue. The cause(s) are unknown.

FLARE   A sudden increase in RA symptoms.

GENE   A specific segment of DNA carrying the code for a specific protein.

GENE THERAPY   Putting genes into a person's cells with the intention of alleviating a gene-based disease.

GENETIC DISEASE   A disease caused by specific genes, e.g., cystic fibrosis, sickle-cell anemia.

GENETIC ENGINEERING   Manipulation of genetic material to alter the genetic traits of cells or organisms, e.g., adding genes to an animal to increase its growth rate.

GENETIC TRANSFORMATION To change an organism genetically by adding new DNA to it.

GLOBULIN The fraction of the blood proteins that contains the antibodies.

GLUCOSAMINE One of the chemicals present in cartilage.

HLA The human leukocyte antigen system—a set of genes that make (MHC) proteins, which mark each individual as chemically unique.

HISTAMINE A substance in the body that expands capillaries and constricts smooth muscle, such as in the lungs.

HUMAN GENOME In an individual, one complete set of twenty-three human chromosomes.

HYPOTHESIS An assumption not yet proven by experiment or observation. The assumption is made for purposes of testing its accuracy.

IMMUNE SYSTEM The complex of cells and chemicals that defends the body against foreign substances, such as bacteria or viruses.

IMMUNE COMPLEX A combination of antigen and antibody, which also may contain complement.

IMMUNITY A state of being resistant to a disease.

IMMUNOGLOBULIN G   The most abundant form of antibody.

INFECTIOUS ARTHRITIS   A form of arthritis caused by disease-causing microorganisms such as bacteria or viruses.

INFLAMMATION   Reactions in which cells and chemicals of the immune system go to a site of infection or damage and interact to produce redness, heat, swelling, and pain.

INTEGRIN   A family of cell surface molecules involved in sticking certain cells together.

INTERLEUKINS   Proteins used for communication between white blood cells.

INTERLEUKIN-1   A proinflammatory cytokine.

INTERLEUKIN-6   A proinflammatory cytokine.

JRA   Juvenile rheumatoid arthritis, with RA onset prior to age sixteen.

JOINT CAPSULE   The fibrous tissue layer surrounding a joint.

KNOCKOUT ANIMAL   An experimental animal in which a certain type of gene has been disabled so that it no longer functions.

LEUKOCYTE   Any type of white blood cell.

LIGAMENT   Strong connective tissue joining bone to bone at joints.

LYMPH NODES   A rounded mass of lymphatic tissue found along the course of lymphatic vessels. Major groups of lymph nodes are found in the armpits, groin, and neck.

LYMPHATIC SYSTEM   A system of thin vessels and lymph nodes. The vessels drain fluid from the tissues of the body, filter it through the nodes, and return it to the bloodstream.

LYMPHOCYTES   Cells, including the T cells and B cells, that make up about 20 to 50 percent of total white blood cells.

MHC   The major histocompatibility complex. Same as the HLA system.

MACROPHAGE   Large mobile cells that pick up particles, including antigens. They can present antigens to T cells, and produce inflammatory chemicals.

METABOLISM   All the chemical reactions that go on inside living organisms.

MEMORY CELL   T cells and B cells that retain the ability to recognize an antigen if it again enters the body. These cells allow a quicker response to the antigen.

MONOCLONAL ANTIBODY   Antibodies made in the laboratory against a specific antigen.

MYCOPLASMA
Bacteria that lack cell walls. Some hypothesize that these bacteria can cause RA.

NSAID
A nonsteroidal anti-inflammatory drug used to reduce pain and inflammation.

NO
Nitric oxide, a gas made by the body's cells. It has many functions, including a role in inflammation.

NATURAL KILLER CELLS
Certain white blood cells that can destroy other cells, such as virus-infected cells or tumor cells.

NEUTROPHIL
A type of white blood cell that can engulf and digest particles.

ORAL TOLERANCE
The natural process of tolerance that the body develops for the antigens in our food that are absorbed through the intestinal wall.

OSTEOARTHRITIS
A disease of the joints characterized by a breakdown of the cartilage and painful, impaired joint function.

OSTEOPOROSIS
A condition of weakened, porous bones most common in the elderly.

PATHOGEN
A microorganism, such as a bacterium or virus, capable of causing a disease.

PANNUS
The destructive overgrowth of the synovial joint lining in RA.

PARENTERAL
Any route other than through the digestive system, e.g., intravenous.

PAUCIARTICULAR JRA
A form of JRA in which generally four or fewer joints are inflamed asymmetrically, that is, if one knee or wrist is affected, the other isn't.

PIPELINE
In pharmaceutical companies, the lengthy process through which products must pass, during which they are tested for their safety and effectiveness.

PLACEBO
Any substance known to be inactive, given to someone to satisfy his or her demand for medicine or used in a clinical trial to compare its effect with that of an active substance.

PLASMA CELL
Formed from a B cell. The plasma cell makes antibodies.

POLYARTICULAR JRA
A form of JRA that affects many joints.

POLYMYALGIA RHEUMATICA
A condition marked by pain in shoulder and hip muscles, and elevated erythrocyte sedimentation rate.

POLYPEPTIDE
A chain of amino acids. Proteins often consist of several joined polypeptides.

PROMOTER
A segment of DNA where an enzyme can attach in order to start the process of copying the message on a particular gene, so that a specific protein can be made.

PROSTAGLANDINS   Chemicals, produced in the body's tissues, that have many effects, including pain.

PROTEINS   Large molecules essential to life. They consist of one or more polypeptide chains of amino acids.

PSORIASIS   A skin disease of unknown cause, with many different forms.

PSORIATIC ARTHRITIS   A form of arthritis associated with psoriasis. The symptoms fluctuate along with those of the psoriasis.

RADIOLOGICAL   Pertaining to radiology, often referring to the use of X-rays.

RECEPTORS   Molecules on cell surfaces that can bind only to specific molecules that may come in contact with the cell.

REFRACTORY   Resistant to treatment.

REMISSION   A period during which symptoms lessen.

RHEUMATIC DISEASE   Any disease that affect connective tissue, e.g., RA, scleroderma, systemic lupus erythematosus (lupus).

RHEUMATOID ARTHRITIS   A systemic autoimmune disease of unknown cause characterized by painful inflammation of the joints and related structures. It may lead to severe joint deformities. Also referred to as RA.

RHEUMATOID FACTOR   An antibody found in many people with RA, and in other diseases as well, e.g., scleroderma, influenza.

RHEUMATOLOGIST   A physician who specializes in rheumatic diseases.

SAARD   A slow-acting antirheumatic drug. The term is synonymous with DMARD.

SCLERODERMA   A disease characterized by a hardening of the skin. It also involves changes in other areas such as the gastrointestinal tract.

SERONEGATIVE   Lacking the rheumatoid factor in the blood.

SHARED EPITOPE   A portion of a gene shared by many people with RA. It may be linked to susceptibility to RA or to its severity.

SINGLE-BLINDED   A clinical trial in which the subjects do not know if they are getting the test substance or an inactive substance.

SJOGREN'S SYNDROME   When associated with RA, marked by decreased saliva and tears.

STEM CELL   A nonspecialized cell that, depending on circumstances, can differentiate into any of the many different cell types in the human body.

STEROID   A large group of chemical substances including the steroid hormones.

STILL'S DISEASE   Another term for systemic onset juvenile rheumatoid arthritis.

SYNGENEIC   Term describing individuals whose tissues are compatible, e.g., twins.

SYNOVIUM   The smooth lining of a joint.

SYNOVIAL JOINT   A flexible joint lined by a synovial membrane.

SYNOVIAL FLUID   Lubricating fluid made by the synovial membrane in a joint.

SYSTEMIC   Pertaining to the whole body.

SYSTEMIC LUPUS
ERYTHEMATOSUS   An inflammatory disease of connective tissue affecting the skin, joints, kidneys, nervous system, and mucous membranes. Also known as lupus or SLE.

SYSTEMIC ONSET JRA   A type of arthritis occurring in children. It is marked by fever, chills, rash, and inflammation of joints and organs.

T CELL   A type of white blood cell that plays a central role in inflammation and is very active in RA.

T CELL RECEPTOR   A protein site on a T cell surface. Each receptor type binds to a specific antigen type.

TH1 CELLS   "Helper" T cells that are proinflammatory.

TH2 CELLS   "Helper" T cells that are anti-inflammatory.

TENDON — Strong fibrous tissue connecting muscle to bone.

TETRACYCLINE — One of a family of antibiotics effective against a wide variety of microorganisms.

THYMUS — A large gland in the upper chest cavity. It is the site where T cells are prepared for their role in the immune system.

TISSUE — A group of similar cells, e.g., muscle or fat tissue.

TRANSCRIPTION FACTOR — An intracellular chemical that binds to a site near a gene and activates the gene.

TRANSGENIC — An organism that has been given functional genes from another unrelated organism.

TUMOR NECROSIS FACTOR-ALPHA (TNF-ALPHA) — An important inflammatory cytokine.

ULCERATIVE COLITIS — An ulceration of the lining of the large intestine.

VACCINE — A small sample of infectious agents or parts of them, rendered harmless and administered in order to induce immunity to those agents, e.g., tuberculosis bacteria or measles virus.

VASCULITIS — Inflammation of a blood or lymphatic vessel.

VECTOR   A carrier. In the case of a DNA, the vector would carry the gene into an organism's cells.

Index